"Our Lords, the Sick"

McGovern Lectures
In the History Of
Medicine and Medical Humanism

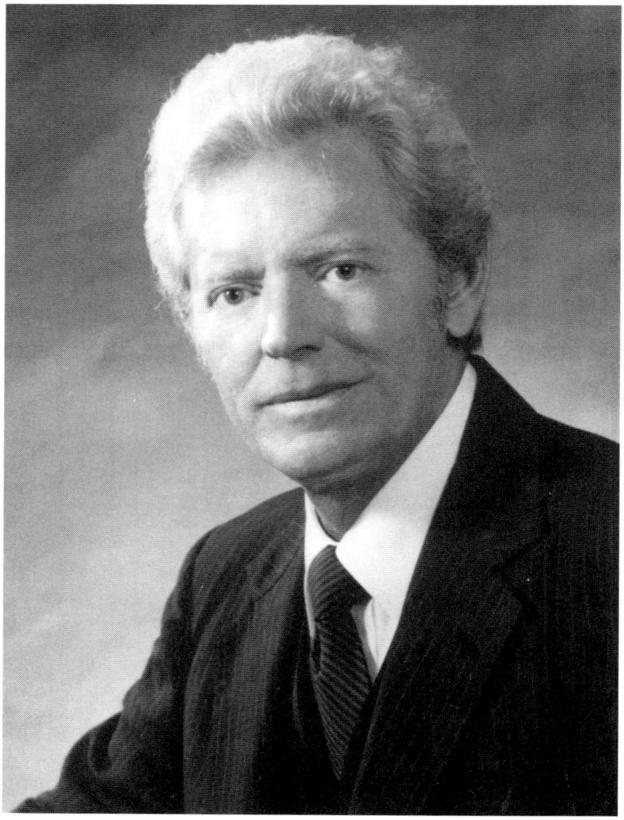

John P. McGovern

"Our Lords, the Sick"

McGovern Lectures
In the History Of
Medicine and Medical Humanism

Edited by
Lawrence D. Longo

With a Foreword by
Philip M. Teigen

KRIEGER PUBLISHING COPMPANY
Malabar, Florida
2004

Original Edition 2004

Printed and Published by
KRIEGER PUBLISHING COMPANY
KRIEGER DRIVE
MALABAR, FLORIDA 32950

Library of Congress Cataloging-in-Publication Data

"Our lords, the sick" : McGovern lectures in the history of medicine and medical humanism / edited by Lawrence D. Longo with a foreword by Philip M. Teigen.—Original ed.
p. cm.
ISBN 1-57524-236-2 (alk. paper)
1. Medicine—History. 2. Humanism. 3. Social medicine. I. Longo, Lawrence D.

R133.6.O97 2005
610—dc22

2004046467

10 9 8 7 6 5 4 3 2

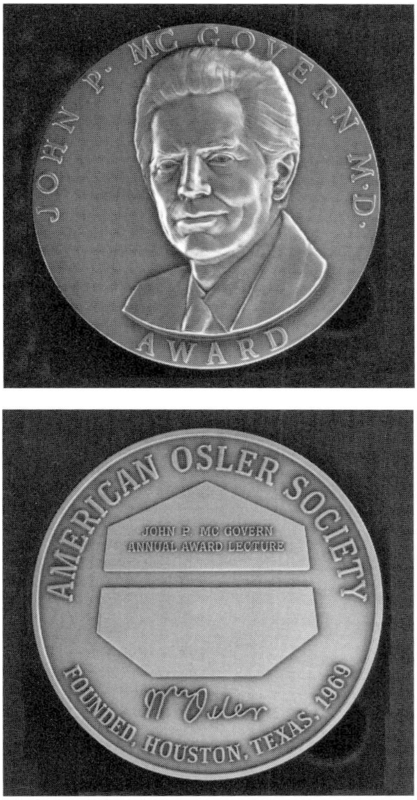

John P. McGovern Medal

Contents

Foreword

"So what?" "Who cares?" say writing teachers to their students when emphasizing the importance of thinking about why and for whom they write. For the same reason it is salutary for writers and readers of medical history to ask themselves these questions also—although not necessarily in such a brusque manner.

Now, members of the American Osler Society—all of them readers and writers of history—might reply that since the Society has been around for three decades, questions about its relevance for medical history are answered already. On the other hand, members of the Society who are enemies of complacency—as Oslerians must surely be—will say that a thirty-third anniversary is just the right time to ask "so what?"

In the 125 years or so that the history of medicine has been studied seriously, three answers to this question have emerged. The first is that medical history is a social good, meaning that with the history of medicine we can recognize and promote important values such as the commitment to individual and public health, clinical prowess, and laboratory innovation. The second answer is that medical history is a political good: it contributes to the larger political effort to prevent medical calamity, to reduce the burden of suffering everywhere, and to heal the sick regardless of creed, class, gender, or origin. The third answer is that medical history is an intellectual good: it explains why things are the way they are.

At the beginning of the twenty-first century, all three of medical history's basic functions are vigorously pursued and—equally important—firmly institutionalized. The American Osler Society (founded in 1969) has become known chiefly for promoting the first good: recognizing, commemorating, and nurturing values important to the medical profession today. The Sigerist Circle (organized in 1990) is focused mainly on the second good: using medical history to enable political changes improving the health and welfare of mankind. The American Association for the History of Medicine (established in 1925) has evolved to focus mainly on the third function: using medical history to advance the understanding of how things really were.

The flourishing of these three institutions and their members is an important source of medical history's interest, strength, and stability. However, in any scholarly enterprise there is a natural inclination to over-specialization. This historiographical reductionism, if unchecked, becomes the enemy of vibrant and fruitful enterprises when, for example, serious biographical or historical writing is dismissed as filiopietistic, hagiographical, or unhistorical. It also occurs when readers condemn historical writing as difficult, dull, and colorless because it uses powerful explanatory theories such as race, class, and gender, or when history without a moral or political "point" is deemed useless or trivial.

The truth of the matter is readers and writers of all three modes of historical writing—social, political, cognitive—need each other. Commemorative history needs professional history to provide factual foundations, politically oriented history needs professional history as a source of models for future action, and professional history needs nonhistorian readers to ensure work that is interesting, readable, and able to be disseminated to the wider world.

Some—but not yet enough—readers and writers of medical history avoid excessive specialization by engaging the entire range of medical-historical subjects in all its modes. Those who don't might well aspire to a greater social, political and intellectual cosmopolitanism, one in which narrow professional loyalties and interprofessional rivalries are replaced with the thoughtful apprehension and appreciation of the entire universe of medical history. Such universalism would not only strengthen the medical history to which we all are committed, it would also acknowledge implicitly the work of William Osler and Henry Sigerist, two of our predecessors most noted for their commitment to the common good.

Philip M. Teigen
History of Medicine Division
National Library of Medicine
Bethesda, Maryland

Preface

Beginning in 1986, the American Osler Society has sponsored an annual lectureship in humanistic medicine, the medical humanities, and the history of the health sciences. Since that time, these orations, supported by an endowment from the John P. McGovern Foundation of Houston, Texas, have been given by prominent medical educators, historians, philosophers, and writers. Yearly, the AOS has published these lectures in a small booklet that is distributed to members of the Society. During twelve years as Secretary-Treasurer of the Society (1988-2000), I edited these and helped see them into print.

Without exception, the authors of these essays have been distinguished scholars. Importantly, the topics and ideas expressed are timeless, and of value to the education of physicians and others in the health science professions, as well as being of vital importance to the meaning of medicine in its broadest sense. Because of their contribution to the life of the mind in medicine, they can be a useful resource for students, physicians, medical educators, and others in the healing arts. Thus, the idea of gathering them into a volume.

Insofar as possible, I have updated the biographical sketches. Also in an attempt to have some consistency in the format, these have been revised, although the text itself is as it was originally presented. Finally, I have endeavored to place the references in a uniform style.

I wish to thank the John P. McGovern Foundation for a subvention to the American Osler Society to assist with this publication. Also, I thank my administrative assistant, Brenda Kreutzer, for her invaluable assistance in verifying the bibliographies, as well as masterful preparation of the manuscript.

Lawrence D. Longo
Loma Linda, California

Introduction

> The Humanities are the hormones, . . . to infect with the spirit of the Humanities is the greatest single gift in education.
>
> William Osler[1]

Great Britain's Classical Association, founded in 1903, is the preeminent group of British scholars in the study of the languages, literature, and civilization of ancient Greece and Rome. Among its objectives is that of promoting classical studies not only among scholars, but in all humanistic education.[2,3] For its president, in general the Association has chosen alternately a classical scholar and a man of wide eminence outside of the classics.[4] As the Association's fifteenth president, William Osler (1849-1919), in May 1919, at its meeting in Oxford, gave his presidential address *The Old Humanities and the New Science*.[5] This was to be his last major oration.

This address was given just six months following the armistice of the Great War, in which he had lost his only son. It is of particular interest, for Osler's challenge to his audience—that of the neglect of an understanding of science by humanists, and a similar lack of *Literae Humaniores* by scientists. Osler admonished "Two things are clear: there must be a very different civilization or there will be no civilization at all; and . . . neither the old religion combined with the old learning, nor both with the new science, suffice to save a nation bent on self-destruction."[6] Paraphrasing Mark Twain [Samuel Langhorne Clemens (1835-1910)] "the so-called Humanists have not enough science, and Science sadly lacks the Humanities."[7]

In making an analogy to the recently discovered importance of the thyroid gland to cellular metabolism, Osler noted the role of the humanities in bringing the student into contact with the great thinkers of the world—"with the dead who never die, with those immortal lives 'not of now or of yesterday, but which always were.'"[8] "The pulse of every student should beat faster" he continued, "as he reads the story of Archimedes, of Hero, of Aristarchus" and others who contributed to our understanding.[9] In this academic celebration consisting of the *crème de la crème* of British classicists, Osler claimed ". . . to have been sailing under false colours," and not to be in ". . . possession of even the traditional small Latin and less Greek." He adjured that he was but an ". . . amateur . . . [among] a body of experts, . . . not an educated man in the Oxford sense. . . . a mere picker-up of learning's crumbs, . . . and . . . a fool among the wise."[10] Nevertheless, in his usual manner, he referred to or quoted close to three dozen philosophers and literary figures from the Greeks to modern times. In this address, Osler drew upon the theme of an essay by the White's Professor of Moral Philosophy, John Alexander Stewart (1882-1948), who in considering the postwar role of Oxford University, stressed the need to establish of a school of *Literae Humaniores*, and that there be no education in "Natural Science without Humane Letters, and no Humane Letters without Natural Science . . ."[11,12]

As William Henry Welch (1850-1934) who happened to be in Oxford at the time, later observed, "Published contributions to knowledge constitute the solid basis of the permanent fame of physicians and men of science."[13] During the past century, the role of the physician in society has evolved dramatically. Initially, he (for most were males) was a clinician who saw the sick, worked with relatively simple tools to make a diagnosis, and then prescribed appropriate treatment. The student's education included the "basic sciences" of biochemistry, microbiology, and physiology. In his clerkship on the wards, he learned to apply this knowledge to understanding disease and its manifold manifestations. In former times, such knowledge may have been sufficient. However, during recent decades, with the enormous increase in knowledge of cellular and subcellular biology, a new era of twenty-first century molecular medicine demands that the healer encompass a much wider body of information. In addition, he or she must assimilate knowledge of bioethics, sociology, anthropology, and related humanities, integrating this in an attempt to develop competent skills and critical judgment. Nonetheless, as in the past, the modern day physician must be primarily a "healer" who "ministers to the sick."

To be more effectual in this role, ideally the contemporary physician, in addition to scientific knowledge, must have a wide appreciation for the history of the profession, a grasp of literature both ancient and modern, and dedication to the patient and the importance of clinical care. Some of these qualities go under the rubric of medical humanism. In referring to William Osler as an embodiment of such a humanistic approach, George T. Harrell (1908-1999), the late Vice-President for Medical Sciences at the Milton S. Hershey Medical Center, The Pennsylvania State University, Hershey, Pennsylvania, noted,

> . . . Osler was recognized as a humanist as well as a superb physician by both his American and British colleagues and friends. He lectured and wrote on philosophy, read voraciously, and collected one of the world's finest personal libraries, meticulously selected to cover

> a wide range of classical and medical fields. Reading of classical or non-medical books was recommended by Osler at bedtime to lessen the tensions of practice and for pure intellectual enjoyment. . . . These efforts can help form a pattern of continuing self-education and improvement as a compassionate physician with true interest in his patients, as was taught by William Osler.[14]

The fabric of medicine is a complex tapestry, with threads of different colors and hues woven together to make the whole. It was, in part, to inject into this milieu more of a perspective of the history of medicine, medical humanism, and Oslerian ideals, as well as to provide a forum for the presentation of ideas from different perspectives, that in 1986 John P. McGovern established the lectureship that bears his name. Since that time, through the generosity of the McGovern Foundation to the American Osler Society, this annual Award Lectureship has been continued. The lectureship makes possible an annual oration dedicated to the life, work, and ideals of Sir William Osler. This includes interests in the interface between the humanities and the sciences—in particular, medicine, literature, philosophy, and history. The lectureship is awarded to a leader of wide reputation who is selected by a special committee of the Society, and is especially significant in that it also stands as a commemoration of Dr. McGovern's own longstanding interest in, and contributions to, Osleriana.

John P. McGovern earned his undergraduate and medical degrees from Duke University. He was greatly influenced by the first dean of the Duke University School of Medicine, Wilburt C. Davison (1892-1972), who had been a student of Osler's at the Johns Hopkins University School of Medicine. Subsequently, McGovern took postgraduate training at Duke and at Yale University School of Medicine. His graduate medical education included Guy's Hospital in London; *L'Hopital des Enfants Malades* in Paris; Children's Hospital in the District of Columbia; and the Boston Children's Hospital. Early academic appointments were at George Washington University, and as a John and Mary R. Markle Scholar in Medical Science at Tulane University. In 1956, Dr. McGovern moved to Houston, Texas where he founded the McGovern Allergy Clinic, which has grown to become the largest of its kind in the United States.

Rich in associations, accomplishments and friends, Dr. McGovern has earned a remarkable *vita*. He remains founder/consultant of the clinic that bears his name. He is a member of numerous honorary and professional societies; is past president of many professional organizations including the American College of Allergists and the American Osler Society; has numerous honorary degrees; and is the author or coauthor of over 200 books and articles. Among many accolades, Dr. McGovern has been honored with the Clemens von Pirquet Lecture and Award; the William A. Howe Award; the Distinguished Service Award, American School Health Association; the Distinguished Achievement Award, Pi Kappa Alpha; and elected as an Honorary Fellow of the Royal College of Physicians, London, England. His record of service includes a Presidential appointment to the Board of Regents of the National Library of Medicine, which he chaired in 1973-1974. In addition to other contributions, he has founded the McGovern Academy of Oslerian Medicine at the University of Texas Medical Branch in Galveston, established the Osler–McGovern Centre at Osler's Oxford home, 13 Norham Gardens, and the John P. McGovern Museum of Health and Medical Science in Houston.

As Jack D. Key, librarian emeritus of the Library of the Mayo Clinic, Rochester, Minnesota, and past-president of the American Osler Society has noted,

> The Award Lectureship serves as an appropriate vehicle for public acknowledgment of Dr. McGovern's American Osler Society related activities and generosity. In addition, it recognizes his commitment to perpetuating the counsels and ideals of Sir William Osler. Subscribing to these, Dr. McGovern has enthusiastically practiced the axiom and example of Osler "We are here to add what we can to, not get what we can from, life."[15]

In a series of articles on medicine in the United States, Lester S. King (1908-2002) pursued the idea of the interconnectedness of history in terms of medical education, biomedical science, the character of medical practice, and biomedical ethics. He compared events in history to the science of ecology—the mutual dependence of a given ecosystem on many parts of a phenomenological network. King concluded,

> The understanding of history depends on comparable circuitous networks of relationship, extending continuously without boundaries. The interration [*sic*] of events is, I believe, an important message of history. Perhaps the study of medical history will induce sympathy for this network approach with its concepts of interpenetration and continuity. These concepts, I suggest, are really the foundation of all of medicine, and not merely of its history.[16]

In our overly complex contemporary society, science and technology are of obvious fundamental importance. Yet, mirroring the two cultures' dichotomy warned of by Osler, our present culture and educational curricula almost guarantee profound scientific illiteracy by the general populace coupled with the disinterest in history, philosophy, and sociology on the part of physicians and scientists. In almost every field, overspecialization leads to tunnel vision. To compound the problem for the busy clinician, finding a balance between the active life and the contemplative life of the mind is not easy. At the 1965 dedication of the new Countway Library, Harvard Medical School Dean, George P. Berry (1898-1986) cautioned, "As we seek to analyze the complex problems of today and look to the promise of tomorrow, we shall do well to profit from the lessons of the past."[17] A number of articles have addressed this idea.[18] As noted by the authors of one of these papers, "to integrate the study of the humanities in medical school is not to provide doctors with a civilized veneer, but to allow them to reach to the heart of human learning about meaning, life, and death."[19]

During recent decades, education in medicine has become ever more fragmented, with emphasis on science and technology. Rather than being seen as a fellow human being with an illness, the patient is viewed as a malady. The physician treats the disease—not the patient. This may result, in part, from medical education being insulated from the humanities. In his 1910 report on medical education in America sponsored by the Carnegie Foundation for the Advancement of Teaching, Abraham Flexner (1866-1959) considered the "Proper Basis of Medical Education" as consisting of not only the biomedical sciences, but stressed the need for the physician to be ". . . an educated man."[20] For too few contemporary physicians, history, philosophy, and other social sciences are woven into the warp and woof of their educational experience. Eric J. Cassel in *The Place of the Humanities in Medicine*[21] has observed,

> Always a concern, early in the post-Flexner era the debate over the proper educational background for physicians resumed, and the tension between humanism and scientism has continued ever since. As Bruer has shown, commissions and reports from the late 1920s to the present era, have championed liberal education over narrow vocationalism. Nonetheless, continuing surveys of medical school requirement testify to the lack of impact of such recommendations.[22, 23]

Some may question the value of a series of orations as compiled in the present volume. However, perhaps we can learn from Montaigne. Michel Montaigne (1533-1592) lived at a time in many ways not too far removed from our own. The late sixteenth century was an age of dissimulation, corruption, violence, and hypocrisy. By definition, his *Essais* were "attempts," "endeavors," and "experiments"—not to achieve absolute truth—but tentatively to explore. While concerned chiefly with the political and religious world, these essays examined almost every aspect of life. Preceding the Enlightenment of the late seventeenth and eighteeth centuries, Montaigne's "attempts" did much to edify his readers, and helped to prepare for the subsequent renaissance in ideas.[24]

As with Montaigne, the present essays are accounts of the individual world view of the writer. They represent interpretations, attempts at understanding. The authors raise questions to help lift our own horizons, to present a broader per-spective on life. They emphasize that while we know much, we understand little. In addition, perhaps they can help us to gain increased self-knowledge in the

Socratic sense, to become more complete human beings, and healers of the highest type.

The diverse set of lectures included in the present volume, then, were conceived to give physicians a broad perspective of medicine and the health sciences, and their relation to the humanities, society, and culture. Each essayist illustrates his or her subject with the importance of social and cultural factors that influenced facets of the history of medicine/medical humanism. The contributors come from differing backgrounds and with points of view—an ethicist, a minister, several internists, two surgeons, a philosopher, several professional historians, and several writers. Six of the authors hold the Ph.D. degree, nine are M.Ds, and two are M.D./Ph.D.s

In his oration to the Classical Association, Osler spoke of the humanities and the sciences being "twin berries on one stem, grievous damage has been done to both in regarding . . . [them] in any other light than complemental."[25] By their life and work, the scholar-authors of these "attempts" have brought fresh light on the humanities and their relation to medicine. They have helped to enlarge the perspective of what medicine is truly about. As with the essays of Montaigne and Osler,[26] this collection is not intended as a text nor as an authoritative final compilation. Hopefully, these commentaries will serve as a stimulus—or invitation—to appreciate the role of the humanities, "the hormones" in medicine, to develop fresh insights and ideas—and to become a contributor to the dialogue of contemporary medical thought. For we who "minister to the sick" in the early twenty-first century, a challenge is to determine who we are and who we wish to be, to broaden our vision, and to catch a glimpse of the great world of the medical humanities, and to appreciate how they may enrich our lives. As such, these essays can help us as healers look inward and reflect on what is of importance for ourselves and for our patients—to practice an ever more humane medicine, filled with respect, compassion, beneficence, and true caring.

References

1. Osler, W. *The Old Humanities and the New Science.* An address before the Classical Association, Oxford, May 16th, 1919. London, John Murray, 1919, pp 14-17. Also published in *Brit Med J* 2:1-7, 1919.
2. Stray, C. (Ed.). *The Classical Association – The First Century 1903-2003* London, The Classical Association, 2003.
3. Osler, W. *The Old Humanities and the New Science.* With Introduction by Harvey Cushing. Boston, Houghton Mifflin, 1920, pp. v-xxii.
4. Ibid., p. vii.
5. Op. cit., #1, entire volume.
6. Ibid., p. 11.

7. Ibid., p. 18.
8. Ibid., p. 15.
9. Ibid., pp. 19-20.
10. Ibid., pp. 3-7, 17.
11. Stewart, J.A. *Oxford after the War & a Liberal Education*. Oxford, B.H. Blackwell, 1919, pp 25, 34.
12. Op. cit., #1, pp. 14, 28.
13. Welch, W.H. Foreword. In: Appreciations and Reminiscences of Sir William Osler, Bart., with a Classified Annotated Bibliography edited by Abbott, M.E. *International Association of Medical Museums and Journal of Technical Methods.* Bulletin No. IX, 1926, p. v.
14. Harrell, G.T. Preface. In: *Medicine and the Comic Spirit*, by Joanne Trautmann Banks, John P. McGovern Lecturer, 1988.
15. Key, J.D. Preface. In: *"Our Lords, the Sick,"* by Albert R. Jonsen, John P. McGovern Lecturer, 1986.
16. King, L.S. The continuity of history. *JAMA* 251:3233-3236, 1984, p 3236.
17. Berry, G.P. The significance of medical history. In: McCord, D.E. (Ed.) *Bibliotheca Medica: Physician for Tomorrow*. Dedication of the Countway Library of Medicine, May 26 & 27, 1965. Boston, Harvard Medical School, 1966, p 28.
18. Davies, R. Can physicians be humanists? *Johns Hopkins Mag* 36:28-34, 1985; Eagle, K.A. Finding humanism in medicine. *Perspect Biol Med* 29:109-114, 1985; Jonsen, A.R. Humanities are the hormones. *Perspect Biol Med* 33:133-142, 1989; Murray, T.J. Why the medical humanities? *Dalhousie Med J* 26:46-50, 1999; Pellegrino, E.D. Educating the humanist physician. An ancient ideal reconsidered. *JAMA* 227:1288-1294, 1974; Pellegrino, E.D. The humanities in medical education. Entering the post-evangelical era *Mobius* 2:133-141, 1982; Risse, G.B. The role of medical history in the education of the 'humanist' physician: A reevaluation. *J Med Educ* 50:458-465, 1975; Robinson, R.R. and F.T. Billings. Some reflections on humanism in medicine. In: Rabin, D. and P. Rabin (Eds.), *To Provide Safe Passage: The Humanistic Aspects of Medicine*. Philosophical Library, New York, 1985, pp 209-221; Self, D.J. (Ed.). *The Role of the Humanities in Medical Education.* Bio-Medical Ethics Program, Eastern Virginia Medical School, Norfolk, VA,1978.
19. Charon, R., and P. Williams. The humanities and medical education. *Acad. Med.* 70:758-760, 1995.
20. Flexner, A. *Medical Education in the United States and Canada. Bulletin Number Four. A Report to the Carnegie Foundation for the Advancement of Teaching.* New York, Carnegie Foundaiton, 1910, p. 26.
21. Cassell, E.J. *The Place of the Humanities in Medicine.* Hastings-on-Hudson, NY, Hastings Center, Institute of Society, Ethics, and Life Sciences, 1984.

22. Op. cit., #17, p. 10.
23. Bruer, J.T. Premedical Education and the Humanities: A Survey. Paper prepared for a Conference on the Humanities and Premedical Education. Sponsored by the Rockefeller Foundation, 25 February, 1980.
24. Montaigne, M. *Essays Translated and Introduced by J.M. Cohen.* London, Penguin, 1958; Montaigne, M. *The Essays: A Selection, Translated by M.A. Screech.* London, Penguin, 1995.
25. Op. cit., #1, p. 18.
26. Osler, W. *Aequanimitas. With other addresses to medical students, nurses and practitioners of medicine.* London, H.K. Lewis, 1904.

"Our Lords, the Sick"*

Albert Rupert Jonsen

Dr. Albert Jonsen is *Emeritus* Professor of Ethics in Medicine at the School of Medicine, University of Washington, where from 1987 to 1999 he was Chairman of the Department of Medical History and Ethics. From 1972 to 1987 he was Chief of the Division of Medical Ethics, School of Medicine, University of California, San Francisco. Prior to that, he was President of the University of San Francisco, where he taught in the Departments of Philosophy and Theology. He received his doctorate from the Department of Religious Studies, Yale University, in 1967. His earlier education was at Gonzaga University in Spokane, Washington, and Santa Clara University in California.

The Institute of Medicine, National Academy of Sciences, elected Dr. Jonsen a member in 1980, and he has served twice on its Council. He was Chair of the National Advisory Board on Ethics in Reproduction (1991-1996), and a member of the National Research Council Committee on AIDS Research (1987-1992). He served as Commissioner on the National Commission for the Protection of Human Subjects of Biomedical and Behavioral Research (1974-1978), and on The President's Commission for the Study of Ethical Problems in Medicine (1979-1982). He is a member of the Medical Advisory Panel, Blue Cross-Blue Shield Association (1986-present). Professor Jonsen is a past member of the Educational Commission for Foreign Medical Graduates, of the American Board of Medical Specilaties, and of the National Board of Medical Examiners. He has been Visiting Professor at Harvard Medical School, Georgetown University, The Johns Hopkins Medical School, Maastricht Institute

*Delivered 12 April 1986 at the Sixteenth Annual Meeting of the American Osler Society, San Francisco, California.

for Health Care Ethics, The Netherlands, and Visiting Scholar, National Library of Medicine, National Institutes of Health. In 1999-2000 he was Visiting Professor of Bioethics, Yale University.

Dr. Jonsen's latest book is *A Short History of Medical Ethics* (Oxford University Press, 2000). He is author of *The Birth of Bioethics* (Oxford, 1998), *The New Medicine and the Old Ethics* (Harvard University Press, 1990), and *Responsibility in Religious Ethics* (Corpus Books, 1971). He is co-author, with S. Toulmin, of *The Abuse of Casuistry* (University of California Press, 1988) and, with M. Siegler and W. Winslade, of *Clinical Ethics* (McGraw-Hill, 1988, 4th edition). He is co-editor, with R. Veatch and L. Walters of *Source Book in Bioethics. A Documenatry History* (Georgetown University Press, 1998); with N. Jecker and R. Pearlman, of *Bioethics: An Introduction to the History, Methods, and Practice* (Jones & Bartlett, 1997); with J. Stryker, of *The Social Impact of AIDS* (National Research Council, 1993) and, with J. Fletcher and N. Quist, of *Ethics Consultation in Health Care* (Health Administration Press, 1989). Professor Jonsen has written chapters in over 70 books on medicine and health care, and his articles have appeared in *The New England Journal of Medicine, Journal of the American Medical Association, Journal of Pediatrics, Annals of Internal Medicine, Journal of Infectious Diseases, Bulletin of the American College of Surgeons, Western Jour-nal of Medicine, The Journal of Medicine and Philosophy, Hastings Center Report, Cambridge Quarterly of Healthcare Ethics, Kennedy Institute of Ethics Journal,* and other publications.

Among the honors received by Professor Jonsen are the Annual Award of the Society for Health and Human Values, the Davies Award of the American College of Physicians, The Lifetime Achievement Award of the American Association of Bioethics and Humanities, and a John Simon Guggenheim Fellowship.

On Saturday, June 22, 1911, the morning post brought to 13 Norham Gardens a confidential letter from 10 Downing Street. The missive bore the news that William Osler, Regius Professor of Medicine, had been created baronet, on the occasion of the Coronation of King George V. Several days later, Dr. Osler wrote to a friend, ". . . they have put a baronetcy on me—much to the embarrassment of my democratic simplicity—but it does not seem to make any difference in my internal sensations."[1] One month later, Sir William spoke in Reading, at the unveiling of memorials to the first and last abbotts of the great medieval monastery of that city—a most uncharacteristic appearance for the Regius Professor, but one to which he had been enticed by a physician whose hobby was the history of the abbey. In his address, the new peer said "you see here in stone symbolized the beginning and the end of a great epoch—of a vast movement to the strength of which our wonderful cathedrals and many other superb ruins bear enduring testimony. Marvelous, indeed, was the faith that found expression in such works! Small wonder that the thirteenth had been called the greatest of centuries."[2]

Sir William, in accepting the baronetcy despite his "democratic simplicity," stepped into a medieval tradition. He became a knight, a peer of the realm. He accepted a title and a few prerogatives—though only a few that came to him from one of the most powerful social institutions of our culture, the knighted nobility, an institution that came into being throughout Europe as the Roman Empire fragmented into innumerable duchies and baronies and counties, served by men sworn to fealty to liege lords.

Certainly, Sir William did not identify himself with the customs, ideals, and concepts of the vanished class—indeed, by speaking of his democratic simplicity, he repudiated them. He graciously accepted the empty honor, long shorn of its political or military might. And despite his remark of the occasion of the Reading Abbey ceremony—he was quoting the title of a book by a friend, physician and historian James J. Walsh, *The Thirteenth, Greatest of Centuries*[3,4]—I assume that Osler, like many of his contemporaries, had little respect or love for that era, over which still hung the cloud of the Dark Ages. Sir William was, above all, a classicist both ancient and renaissance and, we can imagine, found something rather extreme, rather grotesque in the gothic.

But I take this entry into the titled nobility more as a symbol than as a significant fact about Osler's life and thought. Sir William was more a peer of medicine than a peer of the realm. He came to prominence at a time when a number of medical men had attained notice among their colleagues and before the public—a notice that paid respect to scientific learning and healing skills but above all to their creation of a distinctive profession, in the modern sense. Educated in universities, authors of scholarly volumes, influential in public affairs, particularly in the relatively recent public health reforms, founders and promoters of the relatively recent public hospitals—these men formed a kind of nobility. They were, in skills and in science, persons of account, far more so than their somewhat frivolous and overbearing predecessors, the jealous and sometimes vicious members of the Royal College. Many of these peers of medicine had been knighted: Sir Arthur Keith, Sir Thomas Lewis, Sir James Mackenzie, Sir Ronald Ross, Sir Thomas Allbutt, whom Osler's close friend, medical historian Charles Singer, called, "the most learned physician of the last 100 years"[5] and above all, the great Lord Lister, Baron of Lyme Regis. In democratic America, Osler had left behind an untitled peerage of equal prestige: Oliver Wendell Holmes, William and Charles Mayo, Walter Reed, William Stewart Halsted, William Henry Welch and the young man who would become his biographer, Harvey Cushing. Sir William and his contemporaries brought to the medical profession a respect it had historically lacked. It still enjoys the trailing clouds of glory.

These peers of medicine also were nobles in their ethics toward their patients. While it is difficult to know with certainty, both because the record is not written and the motives of men cannot be easily read, I have the impression that their ethics were "noblesse oblige." Although we use this phrase with disdain today, it has a noble history. It recalls the moral obligation placed on lords to protect their vassals, or knights to protect the poor and the weak. Power, coming ultimately from God, was to be used for God's favored poor; fealty to a liege was reciprocated by the liege's duty to protect the vassal. An ethic perhaps more honored in the breach—I do not know—but certainly an ideal that made civilization out of chaos.

I estimate that the great physicians of the late nineteenth and twentieth centuries maintained, even unknowingly, such ethics. The opening words of the paradigm book of medical ethics, penned by Thomas Percival in 1803, bear witness in elegant language to the ethic of *noblesse oblige*,

> Physicians and surgeons should minister to the sick, reflecting that the ease, health and lives of those committed to their charge depend on their skills, attention and fidelity. They should study, in their deportment, so to unite tenderness with steadiness, and condescension with authority, as to inspire the minds of their patients with gratitude, respect and confidence.[6]

Those words were incorporated into the Code of Ethics of the American Medical Association and stood unchanged from 1847 to 1912; their spirit lived long afterward. I am puzzled somewhat by the rarity of Sir William's allusions to the duty owed towards patients. What we call "ethical problems" are almost unseen in his voluminous writing, as best I know, nothing, for example, like the reflections on truth-telling by his distinguished younger contemporary, Richard Cabot of Harvard. Yet everywhere there is a sense of the Hippocratic obligation "to benefit and, at least, to do no harm." There is a sense, and occasional words, that reflects an attitude of courtesy, respect, kindness. Certainly, there is the sense of dedication to the cure and comfort of the sick, even when it entailed, as it often did in those days, some personal risk.

The ethic of noblesse oblige, despite its somewhat antique formulation and dated sentiments, is, indeed, a noble one. It is rigorous in its demands and gracious in its effects. Those who lived by it did much good. What can be said in criticism of this ethic? It is difficult to criticize it without seeming either a cynic or so morally fastidious as to be foolish. Yet, I dare to do so in the name of an important principle, one which, if adopted, leads to a number of implications quite different than the principle of noblesse oblige.

As I noted Sir William's acceptance of a medieval honor, taken as a symbol, my criticism also turns on a medieval fact, taken as a symbol. Sir William most probably knew of the Knights Hospitallers of St. John of Jerusalem—indeed, he may have been inducted as an honorary member of the English Priory, although I can find no evidence of this. However, he probably paid little attention to the history of that religious-military order and knew little of its practices.

Founded in Jerusalem at the end of the eleventh century, its original purpose was to provide hostels for pilgrims to the Holy Land and to care for the sick among them. It established at Jerusalem, Acre, and other places on the route from Eastern Europe to Palestine, institutions that were the precursors of the modern hospital. The famous Hotels-Dieu, which were the more immediate modern predecessors of our modern hospitals, were modelled on the Hospitals of the Knights of St. John.[7]

Within one hundred years of the founding, the order had assumed military duties as well, for it became obvious that the routes of pilgrimage needed to be protected against Moslem incursions. Many local Christian rulers deeded to them frontier castles and, not a century old, the Hospital became a mighty military force. They never abandoned their care of the sick, but this work of mercy became subordinate to the vast military and naval apparatus. The Knights themselves, who were vowed religious, with obligations to celebrate the Divine Office in choir and to live in celibacy and poverty, became soldiers and, in the course of time, it appears that the virtues of religion were overwhelmed by the power and glory of military life.

Still, to the end of the reign of the Knights, which came at the fall of Malta to the Turks in the mid-sixteenth century, the brothers maintained their dedication to hospital work: it remained the soul of their community. Every brother, at his induction into the Knights, recited the vow found in the earliest rule of the Order.

> The brethren of the Hospital should serve our Lords, the sick, with zeal and devotion, as if they were serfs to their Lords. [Rule of 1181]

The Rule again says,

> How should Our Lords, the sick, be received and served? When the sick man shall come to the hospital, let him be received thus: let the Holy Sacrament be given him and afterwards let him be carried to bed and served there as if he were a lord. [Rule of Blessed Raymond, c.1150]

Centuries later, the leaders of the Hospital continue to proclaim,

> We make a promise which no other people make, promising to be the serf and slave of our lords, the sick. [Chapter of 1301]

The rule bears witness to this dedication in many ways: the sick were to be served food before the brothers, were to eat off silver plates, were to be given white bread, were to have first call on bedding. "Our Lords, the sick, shall each have their own sheets and coverlet, broad and long, as well as a gown and slippers to go to the latrine." "Our Lords the Sick who die in the hospital, if they have shirts and breeches, shall be buried in the same." [Chapter of 1301] The revenues that supported the hospitals were not to be diverted to other purposes. In 1296, the officers of the Hospitals complained that the Masters had been spending improperly the resources "that should have been spent for the benefit of our Lords the Sick, to sustain them and the poor."[8]

I am sure many of the brothers left the chapel and rode off to war where they killed and maimed, as did all other knights. I am sure that, corrupted by money and power, they, like many other churchmen, made a mockery of their vows of celibacy and poverty. Yet, in those words, "My Lords, the Sick," they left to all subsequent medicine a precious heritage. They introduced, in antique language, the obligation to serve the sick regardless of risk or cost, a duty unknown to Hippocratic medicine.[9] They placed themselves at the command of those whom they treated; they subordinated, in principle, their ease and their convenience, to the patients whom they received into the Great Hospitals at Jerusalem, Acre, Cyprus and elsewhere.

It is important to realize the meaning, to a medieval man, of an oath, "to be the serf and slave of our Lords the Sick." The Knights of the Hospital, who were often born and bred of the nobility, knew clearly the social position of the serf. The serf simply had no rights and certainly had many and onerous duties. Will Durant lists seventeen obligations of the serf to the lord, ranging from taxes in money to days of labor in corvee and even including the infamous *jus primae noctis,* in which the serf's right to sleep with his bride had to be redeemed by money. While in fact, as Durant says, the actual life of the serf may not have been as terrible as we imagine it, it was one defined in terms of obligations and not in terms of rights or privileges.[10]

What, then, is the difference between an ethic of *noblesse oblige* and the ethic of dedication as a serf to the sick? What relevance does it have to modern medicine and contemporary practitioners? I suggest that modern medicine must ask itself whether its practitioners are a peerage in the fashion of Sir William and his colleagues, or a nobility like the Knights of the Hospital? But isn't this a foolish suggestion? Why should modern physicians think of themselves as a peerage or a nobility at all? Is not such a metaphor outmoded, indeed even outrageous?

I would not dismiss it too quickly. First, the profession is still held in high honor, even though its prestige has slipped somewhat. Second, it is still a profession held by an obligation to compliance and to service—it alone among the professions still honors an Oath. In these features, it is somewhat like a nobility. But even more, it is held to act in concert as a barrier, a wall of protection, against the ravage of illness in individuals and in society. In this, it acts as did the medieval nobility, protectors of the realm. Sir William recognized these duties, saying, "the physicians' challenge is the curing of disease, educating the people in the laws of health and preventing the spread of plagues and pestilence."[11]

However, the knights of the realm and the knights of the Hospital differ. The former hold power and bend to protect the poor; the latter, in principle, hold no power and vow to serve the poor. In this is the modern lesson. The nobility of medicine has, in the last century, attained great power: the profession's monopoly has created great institutions and controls a vast economy. Their control lies, not in the sword but in the prescription and in admitting privileges. However, in recent years, that power is being eroded. The government, the insurance companies, the courts and legislators have whittled away at that power.

Now, as medicine begins to feel embattled, will it fight, as did the nobility of the *ancien regime* during the age of revolution, to preserve power and privilege? Will it turn, as did those same nobles, from protecting the poor, to protecting themselves and their status? The ethic of *noblesse oblige* falters when the power of the noble is attacked. It is a powerful ethic only when its adherents are safe. Recall that the Declaration of the Rights of Man declared that the Revolution had abolished the feudal state, and with it not only its dominance, but its ethic of *noblesse oblige*.

The dedication of the Knights of the Hospital to "Our Lords, the Sick" is quite different. It sees the relationship not as a spill-over of power, a "trickle down" ethic, a condescending compassion, flowing from power, but as a commitment of all one's energy to those who have no energy. Institutions are constructed to empower the powerless, and those who build and guard them are vigilant lest the institution serve their ends rather than the goal of healing and helping. They are even willing to make personal sacrifice so that this work goes on. When the institution is threatened they rally around their sick rather than around their treasury.

These are, I admit, exaggerated images, yet behind the rhetoric lies a real challenge: at a time when the genuine nobility of medicine, a nobility that arises from the science and compassion of men like Sir William, is compromised and threatened from within and without, at a time when many of medicine's younger practitioners either have forgotten, or have never learned, the ethic of noblesse oblige, the choice of an ethic is crucial. Beyond choice lies the continued commitment to an ethic. The Knights of the Hospital gradually fell away from their primordial ethic. They became the builders of fortresses and navies; they amassed a wealth that made them objects of envy to kings and popes. They ended their long history (though they still exist as an honorary and charitable society) as men of power and military might, who eventually fell before the onslaught of mightier power. The parallel to modern medicine is not, I think, too far-fetched. If it is to survive as a service, inspired by humane concern, it must choose its ethic and remain faithful to it. I am suggesting that the ethic of Our Lords the Sick is worthy of remembrance in these latter days. I hope Sir William, peer of medicine, would agree with me.

References

1. Cushing, Harvey *The Life of Sir William Osler,* Oxford, Clarendon Press, 1925, Vol. II, p. 275.
2. Ibid., p. 281.
3. lbid., pp. 391, 522.
4. Walsh, James. *The Thirteenth, Greatest of Centuries,* New York, Catholic Summer School Press, 1907.
5. Singer, Charles. *A Short History of Medicine.* Oxford, Oxford University Press, 1962, p. 626.
6. Leake, Chauncey. (Ed.), *Percival's Medical Ethics,* Huntington, New York, Krieger, 1976, p. 71.
7. Hume, Edgar. *The Medical Work of the Knights Hospitallers of St. John of Jerusalem.* Baltimore, Johns Hopkins Press, 1940.
8. Riley-Smith, Jonathan. *The Knights of St. John in Jerusalem and Cyprus.* New York, Macmillan, 1976, p. 331.
9. Edelstein, Ludwig. *Ancient Medicine.* Baltimore, Johns Hopkins Press, 1967, pp. 319-348.
10. Durant, Will. *The Age of Faith.* New York, Simon and Schuster, 1950, pp. 555-558.
11. Bean, Robert Bennett and Bean, William Bennett (Eds.). *Sir William Osler's Aphorisms, From His Bedside Teachings and Writings.* Springfield, IL, Charles C. Thomas, 1968, #90, p. 63.

To Humane Medicine: Back Door or Front Door*

Edward Janavel Huth

Edward J. Huth is a well-known medical leader, practitioner, teacher, writer and editor. From 1971 to 1990, he served as Editor of the *Annals of Internal Medicine*, American College of Physicians, Philadelphia, Pennsylvania. From 1991 to 1994, he edited the *Online Journal of Current Clinical Trials,* an electronic journal, for the American Association for the Advancement Science.

A native of Philadelphia, Doctor Huth received a B.A. degree from Wesleyan University where his heavy engagement with courses in critical literary analysis and creative writing foreshadowed the evolving of his medical career into the editorship of the *Annals* . . . . After receiving the M.D. degree from the University of Pennsylvania, he trained in internal medicine at that institution's hospital. In the years before his entering editorial work for the *Annals* he collaborated with J. Russell Elkinton at the University in the clinical investigation of potassium deficiency, mechanisms for renal acidification, and the genetics of, and functional disorders in, renal tubular acidosis. His academic posts have included professorial appointments at both the School of Medicine and School of Veterinary Medicine, University of Pennsylvania, and the Medical College of Pennsylvania.

In 1971 Doctor Huth succeeded Doctor Elkinton as Editor of *Annals of Internal Medicine*. He broadened his dedication to many aspects of medical writing and publishing through serving as chairman of the committee that prepared the 4th and 6th editions of the style manual published by the Council of Biology Editors, as a member of the Board of Regents of the National Library of Medicine, and

---

*Delivered 12 April 1987 at the Seventeenth Annual Meeting of the American Osler Society, Philadephia, Pennsylvania.

as a founder of the International Committee of Medical Journal Editors (the "Vancouver group"). His other national activities related to the intellectual and ethical foundations of medical writing and to publication style have included participation in activities of the American Medical Writers Association, the Council of Biology Editors (now the Council of Science Editors), the American National Standards Institute, the European Association of Science Editors, and UNESCO. These activities provided the basis for his two books, *How to Write and Publish Papers in the Medical Sciences* (1982); *Medical Style and Format: An International Manual for Authors, Editors, and Publishers* (1987); and for his contributions to *Conflicts of Interest in Industry-funded Clinical Research* (1996); and *Medicine in Quotations* (2000).

Doctor Huth is a Master of the American College of Physicians, and a Fellow of the Royal College of Physicians of London.

Not being a member of your society, I cannot even guess what inner needs bring each of you to your meetings. If your needs are to come together once a year at the shrine of Saint William and worshipfully fondle the biographic equivalents of shreds of his shirts, hairclippings, or other relics of fact, I shall disappoint you. I know little about Osler, but I do know more than some of our contemporary students. About 15 years ago at the height of problems with thefts of books from medical school libraries, the librarian at Penn posted a sign one day at the check-out desk: "Osler did not steal library books." The sign had not been up 10 minutes when a student stopped by and asked, "Who is Osler?"

Indeed, who is Osler as he lives in our history and, particularly, how is his life relevant to teaching and practicing humane medicine? One of your most eminent members, George Harrell, has given some answers in his paper on Osler's practice,

> The small amount of time he spent with his own hospitalized private patients is commented on repeatedly over the years, especially for patients, without advanced organic disease. On other patients with interesting disease problems, he would make repeated visits for teaching.
>
> He spent a short time with private patients[,] coming in and out of the room quickly so that patients frequently complained that they did not have time to talk to him or to retaliate to his remarks.[1]

But in contrast,

> He had an unusual facility to make all patients feel that he was interested in them as persons, whether they were on the public wards or on the private pavilion.

The apparent paradox may be accounted for by another of Harrell's assessments,

> He stressed meticulous clinical observation with emphasis on diagnosis and pathogenesis of disease. Laboratory findings were a strong point in the teaching, but definitely were secondary to observation.

"Observation" is the keyword. We are pleased as patients when our needs are truly seen, and Osler's patients may have felt themselves truly seen as persons from his closely inquiring into the details of their illness and thoroughly examining their bodies.

Why should we be concerned today about humane medicine? Is this a more worthy topic today than it would have been in Osler's day? Is medicine less "humane" than it was then? What is "humane" medicine?

All around us are evidences that our society has lost some confidence in medicine as a public service.[2-4] That loss could be due to many different causes and some may be well beyond our control. One expert on effects of the public media has pointed out[3] that television often portrays physicians so idealistically that real physicians fail against the image. Certainly in some surveys of public opinion[4] patients have complained of how they are seen and cared for. Ironically some of this dissatisfaction may stem from the efficiency with which we reach highly accurate diagnoses by rushing the patient off for one of the new almost incredible imaging procedures rather than taking a detailed history at length. This apparent decline in confidence in our capacity for humane care is seen by some keen observers who are not of, but are close to, our profession. A good example is Charles Odegaard, a humanist who has come to know us[5] from his seat in such bodies as the Millis Commission and the Board of Directors of the Clinical Scholars Program run by the Robert Wood Johnson Foundation. Some groups within the profession imply by their actions that they too perceive a decline in confidence in our humaneness; note the great response of the American Board of Internal Medicine represented by its several reports on "humanistic qualities in the internist."[6,7]

If the apparent decline in confidence in medicine is due to a feeling by today's patients, unlike Osler's patients, that we do not see them as persons, perhaps we can find remedies for that defect. I am not sure that we can. Impersonality runs through much of our huge and complex society; I am struck with how often voices in our public media refer to men and women as "people," not as persons. In our increasingly crowded world too many of us do not see the difference between *populus* and *persona*.

How does the patient want to be seen?

Patients are men and women. Patients, like the rest of us, have a view of themselves and of the world around them that has been shaped by their lives as infants and children. The most ancient memory we carry is being cared for in the mother-child dyad. That memory is a frame through which much of our view of others around us must pass;—Dinnerstein, a psychologist who has dissected the problem of dependency[8] more thoroughly than anyone else I know of, puts it thus,

> Few of us ever outgrow the yearning to be guided as we were when we were children, to be told what to do, for our own good, by some one powerful who knows better and will protect us. Few of us even wholeheartedly try to outgrow it.

But the desires go beyond being guided, being told what to do. Consider these questions.

Do you understand me?
Will you help me?
Will you stick with me?
Will you always care for me?
Will you take advantage of me?
Will you always do the right thing for me?

These are questions all children would probably put to their mothers if they could fully phrase their feelings. And the questions emerge in later dyads; these questions are likely to be put, or implied, to a prospective wife or husband. In fact these questions are borrowed and slightly adapted from a paper published recently in the *Canadian Medical Association Journal,*[9] "Our patients' seven unspoken questions." I cannot argue here that these are indeed questions patients have in their minds when they see us, but I point out that some of them are clearly reflected in one classic document that defines, among other matters, what we owe patients in our contracts with them, The Hippocratic Oath.

Among these questions, one, the first, seems to me to be the main question to be asked in assessing whether a physician's care is humane or not. (The term *humane* is not really a satisfactory adjective for the kind of medicine I think we have in mind with "humane medicine." The phrase suggests a possible alternative, inhumane, and there is much care that while not humane in the sense of the phrase is certainly not *inhumane*—unfeeling, brusque, impersonal, or cursory, perhaps, but not inhumane. "Humanistic medicine" is not right either; it implies to me a kind of care embroidered with threads of consciously acquired culture rather than the careful care given by one very human physician to a very human patient.)

"Do you understand me?" This is the patient's first assessment of the physician. The question runs far beyond such simpler questions as "Did you listen to my complaint and do you know what my symptoms are?" It implies a long string of other questions that may not be directly linked to the questions weighed by the physician as he thinks about what disease or disorder or injury the patient brings to the encounter. "Has the physician sized up the relative importance to me of my symptoms? Has the physician accurately gauged the strength of my anxiety, my depression, my confusion, my longing? Does the physician know the limits to the care I can get at home? Does the physician know the limits of my financial resources?" And the questions can run further. I do not mean to imply that most patients always have all of these questions at the front of their minds; they probably do not.

The patient's second question, "will you help me," necessarily implies that the patient expects the help to be tendered by the physician will be properly shaped by the understanding acquired by the physician in accord with the patient's first expectation. Care that satisfies the patient as far as circumstances permit in response to these two questions may be what we call *humane medicine*.

How can we educate and train physicians likely to practice medicine that is "humane" thus defined?

One method is implied by what I presume is a motive behind the annual meetings of your society: If one is educated in the shadow of a model physician, one may move in his steps, the modeling effect. The humane clinical teacher sets out by example a pattern for how to behave humanely. The key term here is *pattern*. But in a particular clinical encounter how does the physician conduct himself if the pattern does not include a picture of a problem? The modeling process is defective when it does not convey operating principles that become working tools for the follower. Indeed, the modeler may have simply worked with a genetically determined package of traits and not on principles. The follower fails when he or she was not born with these traits; perhaps Osler was such a "modeler" and touched followers with his traits while not conveying to them explicit principles for conduct with patients. We can yearn to be like him but if we are not made of the same biological stuff, we may not become even third-rate imitators. This view certainly betrays my conviction that most of our behavior is likely to be genetically determined, a view that is unpopular with educators. Our phenotypes may be shaped in part by education, and one of my later proposals rests on this premise, but the genotype is probably more critical. This view does raise the question of whether we might select medical students for the right behavioral genotypes, certainly a heretical question.

A second kind of proposal for training the humane physician comes from persons thoroughly educated in one of the disciplines known some years back as "the humane letters": the literatures of English, of the other modern languages, and of Latin and Greek. The proposition in general is that medical students or physicians-in-training can be led to be more sensitive to the human condition, and hence to the plight and needs of the patient through the reading, analysis, and discussion of literature, both prose and poetry. I can not recapitulate the argument for this proposal here; it has been well developed by numerous spokesmen. Perhaps the most developed and persuasive argument is that by Eric Cassell[10] in *The Place of the Humanities in Medicine*. In brief, the argument is that literature shows us the human plight, that medical students can be led to see that plight through literature, and that such knowledge tells us in advance what we will find in patients. Can literature really change us that deeply? I am skeptical. My skepticism comes, I know, from my own experiences. I feel that in the arts one is ready to really see or to really hear or one is not. I remember clearly the first symphonic concert I heard, when I was a freshman in high school. I heard for the first time, among other works I still remember, the Beethoven Fifth Symphony. No one had told me what to hear and how to hear it but that first hearing was like a light's being turned on in a dark room. Nothing I could have been told could have prepared me for the effect; something already in me prepared me to hear. Is anyone moved by literature who has not already been moved by experience? Or who does not already have some innate capacity to be deeply touched by the particular way words not usually charged with deep feeling are put together so as to give them meaning beyond what they usually carry? Consider the famous poem by Emily Dickinson, number 650 in the collection by T. H. Johnson.[11]

Pain—has an element of blank—
It cannot recollect
When it begun— or if there were
A time when it was not—
It has no future—but itself—
Its infinite contain
Its past—enlightened to perceive
New Periods—of pain.

Perhaps no other writer has described pain more powerfully or precisely, but how many students in their twenties will grasp all that that poem says and implies? It presents its own obstacles to comprehension, its quirks in grammar, its quirks in punctuation. Grasping all of its essence calls for both a grasp of the devices represented by its grammatical quirks and the reader's having lived through some pain of duration or some years of caring for persons in relentless and unrelievable emotional or physical pain. Probably the more important point is that literature usually tells you its message but patients often cannot convey what physicians need to know if they would know the whole person of the patient.

What might be a third means of training "humane" physicians?

I go back to a phrase in Harrell's account of Osler in his practice: "meticulous clinical observation." I emphasize "meticulous" and "observation." These terms carry the essence of the old saw: "To be a good doctor you don't have to be smart but you have to be thorough." But Osler is probably not a paradigm for what many of today's patients would regard as the thorough physician, the physician who sees all of the patient's needs, and I emphasize "all needs." His shortcoming by today's standards is clear enough in Harrell's telling us of patients who complained that he spent too little time with them; this is still a frequent complaint of patients. "Seeing the whole patient" implies knowing the patient's values, yearnings, weaknesses, resources—the whole range of what makes up one's person.

Do we train our medical students adequately in how to see fully the person who is the patient, not only the "medical" facts but the whole fabric into which the "facts" are set? Seeing the whole person is an awesome skill; indeed, no one ever sees the *whole* person, not even by the end of a lifetime together with an intensely devoted spouse. But to me this is the essence of "humane" medicine, and I do not see that this proposition informs today the design of the medical curriculum in even the best of our medical schools, except perhaps the present experimental curriculum at Harvard. The training that would be needed would have to run far beyond the usual present curricular content on history-taking.

Sometimes the problem of educating physicians to see the whole person has been dodged by claiming that one cannot teach the "art" in the "art and science of medicine." I have come to dislike thoroughly that phrase, "art and science." "Art" implies an inborn skill, an intangible skill that cannot be dissected into what makes it up. The "art" of medicine is a skill I believe can be analyzed, defined, and taught. To the extent that the skill can be observed closely, detailed as to its components, defined for its execution, and systematically applied, it is science and not "art."

Nevertheless how to train the medical student to "see the whole person" is an awesome problem. The problem is in part due to the age of the student. What medical students know themselves well enough at their age to be able to see the whole person in someone else—McWhinney has quoted in one of his recent papers a passage[12] that nicely sums up the problem,

> Mature awareness is possible only when I have digested and compensated for the biases and prejudices that are the residue of my personal history. Awareness of what presents itself to me involves a double movement of attention, silencing the familiar and welcoming the strange. Each time I approach a strange object, person or event, I have a tendency to let my present needs, past experience or expectations for the future determine what I will see. If I am to appreciate the uniqueness of any datum, I must be sufficiently aware of my preconceived ideas and characteristic emotional distortions to bracket them long enough to welcome strangeness and novelty into my

> perceptual world. This discipline of bracketing, compensating, or silencing requires sophisticated self-knowledge and courageous honesty.

How many medical students enter medical school equipped with this maturity?

Is one solution to preparing practitioners with the needed emotional foundations for a full and clear view of patients' needs some better method with which we select students for admission? I cannot review here the premises with which we decide who gets into medical school. Are motives for entering medicine good predictors of who will be humane physicians? The literature on motives and their value for selection is scanty. The overt motives for entering medicine have been described in some formal studies of which that by Rogoff[13] may still be the most complete. But we know little of underlying emotional motives. They probably little resemble the usually stated motives and may have far more to do with what kind of physician one becomes. Lawrence Kubie, a one time psychiatrist at Yale and a sharp observer of the emotional structure of physicians in academic medicine, commented thus.[14]

> When a youth decides to become a doctor, a lawyer, a businessman, or an artist, the decision is not made ... out of a deep introspective knowledge of himself and of how he would fit into the lifework he has chosen.

Some of the evidence for a primacy of deep-seated, emotional motives for entering medicine comes from biographical data. One good example comes from the life of Willa Cather, the great American novelist in the literature of the American Midwest. In a recently published biography of Cather, Sharon O'Brien"[15] closely describes Cather's strong desire in adolescence to become "William Cather" and to study medicine. Her desire appears to have stemmed from her seeing her mother, and hence women in general including herself, as weak. She saw her mother roused from what was probably a neurotic asthenia[16] by a competent, forceful male practitioner who became for a while her ideal. Medicine as a vocation could give her the strength she craved in the face of seeing women, and particularly herself, as weak. But could Cather, if she had entered medicine with such a motive, have tolerated the "weakness," the dependency of patients, which she would have despised in herself?

I must concede we have little evidence that unconscious motives which lead physicians to enter medicine limit their capacities to see the "whole person" and deal adequately with the patient's dependencies. But physicians do grow up with the same dependency needs and defenses against them as other persons. We are not exempt from the human condition. If we have those needs and cannot consciously tolerate them as adults, can we tolerate them in our patients so that we can adequately serve them in accord with their needs? If we do not have a deep awareness of "the biases and prejudices that are the residue" of our personal histories, can we see patients clearly?

We can not realistically expect medical schools to identify in their applicants the emotional matrixes out of which came decisions to enter medicine. Even if they could, would they be able to predict what emotional matrixes in students at entry would best enable them much later in practice to adequately care for others? What medical schools could do, however, would be to train students from the very first week of school in close observation of patients, in seeing patients entire—social, cultural, economic, emotional. But such training would have to include training them to observe themselves, to see how and when their own weaknesses cripple their capacity to truly see patients and to shape care accordingly.

The problem of educating to be able to "see the whole person" and then be able to provide carefully informed by what they see and know, including what they know about themselves, has not been ignored. The Society for Research and Education in Primary Care Internal Medicine has a group of members intensely devoted to "the medical interview and related skills" and their views, recommendations, and persuasions are carried regularly in a newsletter, *Medical Encounter*. A few medical schools have programs for the development of these skills at the residency level. But very few medical schools in the United States or Canada begin training their students at the very beginning of their education in the skills of seeing the "whole person" and translating that view into what the patient needs as circumstances and resources permit. And I do not know that any schools systematically train students through their four years in self-observation.

If this judgment as to what medical schools should do to prepare their students to become truly humane physicians is correct, could our schools revise their curricula to do what is needed? I doubt it. The political problems in attempts at thorough and rational revision are enormous. We all know the special pleading and self-serving arguments that arise from basic-science departments if it is proposed that medical schools exist first and mainly to train practitioners to care for the ill and the injured. Even if this premise is accepted there are the wasteful territorial claims to curriculum from narrow clinical specialists that crowd out possibilities for greater curricular concentration on skills that are vital to good care in any specialty. The problem of getting out of present orthodoxies in curriculum is nicely illustrated by the widely-known and cited General Professional Education of the Physician and College Preparation for Medicine (GPEP) report.[17] Assembled from the views of a large number of medical academicians, the report does specify some details for clinical training in skills relevant to truly knowing patients and their families but holds to the conventional wisdom that this is mainly the business of the "clinical years." Unsurprisingly it ignores completely the critical need for physicians' self-knowledge in the patient-physician dyad.

The one influential group that seems to have wrestled more effectively so far with the essence of needs in training the humane physician is a subcommittee of the American Board of Internal Medicine. Its report[7] should be read closely be all medical educators. Unfortunately the Board's influence on training is mainly in residency programs and is unlikely to touch curricular committees largely representing constituencies other than internal medicine.

Perhaps some day in the distant future, universities will come to see that their medical schools themselves have become medical-science universities and that the one-time central purpose of schools of medicine is buried under tons of research enterprises that bring in money and earn distinction but, despite their distant relevance to care of the ill, contribute next to nothing to the central purpose. When the day of that insight arrives, some medical educators may have the sense to reinvent the college of medicine, move the peripheral enterprises to some other locus, and make sure that its dimensions and units are such that it will devote itself efficiently and rationally to preparing physicians for the proper care of the ill. This hope is, I admit, utopian.

References

1. Harrell, G.T. Osler's practice, *Bull Hist Med* 47:545-68, 1973.
2. [Anonymous]. Doctors face image conflict, future regulation hinges on balancing economics and patient confidence now, *Med World News* 28: 12, 14, Apr 13, 1987.
3. [Anonymous]. Physicians' woes are pervasive, *Med World News* 28: 14, Apr 13, 1987.
4. Okrent, O. You and the doctor, striving for a better relationship. *NY Times Magazine*, Mar 29 (Pt 2): 18-9, 21, 92, 94, 1987.
5. Odegaard, C.E. *Dear Doctor, A Personal Letter to a Physician.* Menlo Park, CA, Henry J. Kaiser Family Foundation, 1986.
6. Subcommittee on Evaluation of Humanistic Qualities in the Internist. *Report of Subcommittee on Evaluation of Humanistic Qualities in the Internist.* Philadelphia, American Board of Internal Medicine, 1983.
7. Subcommittee on Evaluation of Humanistic Qualities in the Internist. *A Guide to Awareness and Evaluation of Humanistic Qualities in the Internist.* Philadelphia, American Board of Internal Medicine, 1985.
8. Dinnerstein, D. *The Mermaid and the Minotaur, Sexual Arrangements and Human Malaise.* New York, Harper & Row, 1976, p. 188.
9. Ney, P.G. and Ney, P.M. Our patients' seven unspoken questions. *Can Med Assoc J* 135: 879-880, 1986.
10. Cassell, E.J. *The Place of the Humanities in Medicine.* Hastings-on-Hudson, Institute of Society, Ethics and the Life Sciences, 1984.

11. Johnson, T.H. (Ed.). *The Complete Poems of Emily Dickinson*. Boston, Little, Brown, 1960, p. 323.
12. Keen, S. *To a Dancing God*. New York, Harper & Row, 1970, p. 28. Quoted in: McWhinney, I.R. Are we on the brink of a major transformation of clinical method? *Can Med Assoc J* 135: 873-878, 1986.
13. Rogoff, N. The decision to study medicine. In: Merton, R.K., Reader, G.G., Kendall, P.L. (Eds.). *The Student-Physician, Introductory Studies in the Sociology of Medical Education*. Cambridge, MA, Harvard University Press, 1957.
14. Kubie, L.S. Some unsolved problems of the scientific career. *Am Scientist* 41: 596-613, 1953.
15. O'Brien, S. Chapter 5, Enter William Cather. In: *Willa Cather, The Emerging Voice*. New York, Oxford University Press, 1987, pp. 96-113.
16. O'Brien, S. *Willa Cather, The Emerging Voice.* New York, Oxford University Press, 1987, p. 91.
17. Association of American Medical Colleges. Physicians for the twenty-first century. Report of the Project Panel on the General Professional Education of the Physician and College Preparation for Medicine. *J Med Educ* 59 (11 Pt 2): i-208, 1984.

Medicine and the Comic Spirit*

Joanne Trautmann Banks

Joanne Trautmann Banks became the first full-time professor of literature at a medical school when in 1972 she took a position at the Pennsylvania State University College of Medicine, where she is still Adjunct Professor of Humanities. She now lives in Florida and continues her lecturing, consulting, and writing. Her books include *Literature and Medicine: An Annotated Bibliography* (1975; revised 1982), *Healing Arts in Dialogue,*(1981), and *The Use and Abuse of Literary Concepts in Medicine.* (1986). Outside of medicine, she is best known as the co-editor of the *Letters of Virginia Woolf* (1975), and the sole editor of Woolf's selected letters, *Congenial Spirits* (1989).

George T. Harrell, Vice President for Medical Sciences, Emeritus, The Milton S. Hershey Medical Center, The Pennsylvania State University, has written of Professor Banks,

> At its founding, the new school she joined had determined to emphasize patients as people who had diseases or problems which interfered with their lives and required help. Accordingly, the first full academic Department of Humanities in any medical school was established. The first appointments in religion and philosophy were soon followed by literature. Why literature? The department was placed adjacent to family medicine which was the first clinical department organized, and to function as a basic science. Working together these faculties could help students . . . to focus on influences other than the disease

*Delivered 3 May 1988 at the Eighteenth Annual Meeting of the American Osler Society, New Orleans, Louisiana.

process which might reflect on the acceptance of the illness and compliance by the patient and family with the physician's recommendations. Success in the treatment plan, or achievement of the best possible result, and adjustment to it would require recognition of cultural, religious, educational level and other factors impinging on the patient.

Authors from the beginning of recorded history have been keen observers and interpreters of why people, families, and populations have certain values and behave as they do. The early Greeks recognized and accurately described psychiatric problems and we still use the names given to some. Over the years, writers have described epidemics or the motivation for population movements. The same approach is true with today's authors, playwrights, and poets.

Students are taught by the scientific faculty about inherent biologic variability between individuals and the range between which laboratory data or observations may vary in health and disease. Literature can illustrate similar variability between individuals and their reactions to, and perceptions of, illness, disease, and stresses in family, work settings or societal changes in the real world outside.

Reading of classical or non-medical books was recommended by Osler at bedtime to lessen the tensions of practice and for pure intellectual enjoyment. Dr. Banks has succeeded superbly in meeting our hopes in her teaching and writing as she pioneered in this new field. This lecture illustrates her ability to stimulate students to read literature other than medical, and to think about it. As a byproduct, not as a planned objective, students have learned the need to express themselves more clearly and accurately in their own and patient records, or for any publications, lay or scientific, they may write. Also, they have learned to communicate with patients and families at levels they can understand with a minimum of scientific terms or jargon.

These efforts can help form a pattern of continuing self-education and improvement as a compassionate physician with true interest in his patients, as was taught by William Osler.

Of the many potential values that are engendered by a group such as the Osler Society, devoted to the work of a distinguished person from the past, one, for me, is paramount: the dialogue with the dead. If that idea seems outlandish, please consider that a good deal of our continuing education is, or at least should be, conversation with dead people. I read Virginia Woolf, for instance, to hear her narrative voice while she constructs the world as she perceives it. I speak back to her, saying, "Yes, I see that the world is sometimes like that," or "No, you've not persuaded me on that point." As I read her more carefully, I strive to reach the level of deepest involvement, wherein I ask the Virginia Woolf I now know, "Here's a new proposition; what do you think of it?" And she, in a sense, replies. Thus are the deserving classics kept alive.

I assume that most of you have a similar relationship with Sir William Osler. You exhume his life and values not primarily out of nostalgia or to create a hero, but to speak with him, to test whether or not his ideas resound through the years, and to decide, with each other, how best to continue in his spirit.

I do not know Osler nearly as well as you do. But I have spent the past several months imagining myself in dialogue with him, particularly as the writer of *Aequanimitas*. You remember what he said in that valedictory address to the faculty and students of the University of Pennsylvania. To achieve equanimity in the practice of medicine, Osler declares, physicians should cultivate a "judicious measure of obtuseness" (wonderful phrase, that), but not at the price of hardening the heart. Do not, he goes on to say, expect too much of your patients; after all, they must forgive you too. So: edit out some of the pain as it comes to you, and don't take the human species so seriously as to think they, and you, are an entirely finished product. His third prescription—his best, I think, and the hardest with which to comply—is to tolerate the uncertainty that is everywhere, not only in medicine, but in existence at large.

I want to ask Osler, and you Oslerians, to consider a fourth route to equanimity, one that subsumes the other three. It is simply this: that comedy, properly understood and properly practiced, is a thoroughfare to the peace envisioned by Osler for his colleagues.

But first I want to tell a story. All ideas begin in stories. My close English friend, Nigel Nicolson, has had a varied career, from soldier to publisher to author. In his young manhood he was for a few years a Conservative Member of Parliament. Soon after his election, he was summoned to the office of the Prime Minister, for the Tories were then in power, to hear a word of welcome and direction. The young parliamentarian trembled as he entered the presence of the great Winston Churchill. But Churchill was too busy to notice. He was submerged in the daily barrage of papers, messages, and phone calls. "Bring in this file, bring in that," he boomed at his private secretary, who dutifully kept the piles of documents mounting before the leader. Eventually the secretary ventured to insert, "Mr. Prime Minister, haven't you forgot Rule 6?" Churchill looked up. "Of course," he said in that famous gruff voice. "Rule 6. Quite right." Immediately, the activity ceased, and Churchill turned his attention to his visitor, who, shy as he felt, could not forbear asking, "Mr. Prime Minister, what is Rule 6?" "Rule 6, young man, is Never Take Yourself Too Seriously." And what are the other five rules, Sir?" "There are no other rules!" replied Churchill.

I think that is true. I think that Rule 6 is deeply true. When, as the phrase goes, all is said and done; when we've read all our books; when we've constructed our theories; when we've analyzed our universe; then, at the root of our ability to perceive matters accurately and live successfully, is Rule 6. Thinkers have written volumes on the nature of comedy, but its basis, standing alone, is Never Take Yourself Too Seriously.

Let me suggest a game to you. Try to decide whether you operate *essentially* from a comic or a tragic point of view. Granted that I have not yet fully defined my terms, but, taking Rule 6 as a working definition of comedy, does the comic point of view frame the events in your life? It's often hard to tell. Some very amusing people have a tragic outlook (and serious people, a comic one). Also remember, please, that the tragic mode is a persuasive one. A working definition of tragedy begins with the assumption that the essential truth about life, the one from which all other meaning is derived, is that individuals die—particularly beloved individuals, among whom (perhaps chief among whom) is oneself. It is easy to demonstrate that life is horrid, if not at present in one's own life, then assuredly at a thousand spots around the globe.

If you decide that, even so, yours is not a tragic perspective, do not then assume that it is a comic one. There are several additional styles. Using other terms borrowed from literature, I can discern, for instance, that some people interpret the world not through the largeness of comedy or tragedy, but through middling pathos. The typical disease-of-the-week television movie is built on pathos. Its effects are bought cheaply. The sight of its sufferers hurts us only momentarily, or even pleasantly, and brings no lasting knowledge. It normally ends with an image or moral, meant to inspire. Likewise, the inspirational articles found in the *Reader's Digest* water down the tragic into the pathetic. The articles about, say, a disabled person who has climbed mountains or someone with Down's Syndrome who has become an actor—these articles do not give full force to the fear and suffering that accompany disabilities. In these cases, sentimentality diverts us.

There are people among us whose basic interpretation of events is, to borrow another literary term, melodramatic. Again, be cautioned: it is not always easy to uncover this perspective, even in ourselves. To be sure, when the Sandy Dennis character in Neil Simon's *The Out of-Towners* whines precisely the same "Oh, my God!" in response to events ranging from her husband's mugging to the loss of one of her false eyelashes, we know we are dealing with someone who regards life as melodrama. But physicians who secretly see themselves as heroic saviors, diseases as villains, and patients as requiring rescue, are themselves setting the stage for a melodrama.

I am afraid that pathos operates in the field that broke into medicine twenty-five years ago as thanatology. Fiercely honest in its inception, thanatologists, it seems to me, are increasingly awash in clichés about dying. I'm not surprised. It is superficially easier to view suffering through the lens of pathos than tragedy or, for that matter, comedy. Even melodrama allows us to handle life's terrors faster. But physicians who see pathos or melodrama everywhere have taken a detour around Osler's equanimity. To reach that destination, comedy is required.

Nonetheless, comedy has never been a popular mode. We pay lip service to the value of those who have a sense of humor, but through the ages the majority of humankind have been suspicious of someone who laughs too much. Plato thought laughter morally suspect because it was directed, he said, at those who are comparatively powerless. Aristotle thought only a little more kindly of comedy, but he wrote some influential passages on the subject. It is Aristotle's work on comedy, in fact, which is the murder weapon in the recent intellectual best-seller (if that is not an oxymoron), Umberto Eco's *The Name of the Rose*. Set in a medieval monastery with a rare and valuable library, reached only through a labyrinth, the novel chronicles the mysterious deaths of several monks. It turns out that all the deceased have managed to read Aristotle on comedy. The readers pay for their new knowledge with their deaths, for the librarian, thinking the book dangerous, has smeared its pages with a slow-acting poison. Comedy, he argues, removes fear; it is fear that makes us need God; ergo, comedy removes the need for God. And if we laugh at the sacred, the world will collapse into chaos.

We do not have to agree with Eco's librarian to realize that comedy has great power in our daily and cosmic lives. In medicine, comedy is deeply rooted in at many levels, the most obvious of which is satire. Doctors have been targets for patients, and patients for doctors, with the result that no one looks very heroic. The comedic exchange, however, appears to be necessary. Two things, said Voltaire, are necessary for survival—hope and sleep. No, there are three, said Kant—hope, sleep, and laughter.

Doctors have always been good for a laugh. By the time of the *commedia dell'arte* in the middle ages, the doctor, blundering, short-sighted, and without any efficacious tools, was already a stock figure. He had his most famous incarnation in the 18th century plays of Molère. In *La Malade Imaginaire, Le Mėdecin Malgė Lui*, and *L'Amour Mėdecin*, Molière's doctors regard pompous jargon as their best therapy and sizeable fees as their just ends. In our own century, the buffoonish physicians in George Bernard Shaw's *The Doctor's Dilemma* and Peter Nichols' *Joe Egg* are still speaking language that is not only incomprehensible to ordinary people but also thoroughly insensitive to those people's feelings. "All professions," asserts Shaw in the preface to his play, "are conspiracies against the laity."

Through comedy of this rather broad type, the laity strikes back. It is not difficult to uncover their motivation. After all, even when doctors knew very little science and practiced barbarous technique, they were nonetheless present at human beings' most vulnerable times. Doctors were, and are, frightening, in that they are associated with what most terrifies people—their own pain and deaths. Doctors are powerfully vertical when patients are horizontal. And when doctors cannot make any difference in an illness, patients are angry in direct proportion to the physicians' arrogance. Moreover, they often appear to make a great deal of money from suffering. To create them as figures of fun in our literary comedy is, therefore, an attempt to cut them down to size and control them.

Of course, doctors laugh at patients too, and for some of the same reasons—namely, fear and anger. Younger professionals, especially, use comedy to disguise their fear about handling human welfare so intimately. One of the most common sources for this kind of humor is the gross anatomy lab. Scarcely anyone has ever visited that place without noting that the medical students attempt to match the obscenity of death with the vulgarity of so-called "black humor." Fear operates on a practical level as well: the patient may rise up and sue me, the doctor thinks, or, worse yet, make me feel incompetent. Laughter keeps such a patient under control. When a patient returns again and again with a complaint that is due to his or her noncompliance with medical advice or to hypochondria, the doctor may likewise respond with humorous stereotyping to handle the inevitable anger or frustration: "I've just seen the hundredth 'Sick, Tired, and Dizzy' of the week." Doctors laugh in order to contain their compassion (as in Osler's "judicious measure of obtuseness"), and thereby prevent paralyzing identification with the sufferer. Sometimes they invent comedic turns simply because they are bored by, for instance, removing the gall bladders of "Fat, Flatulent, and Fortyish Females." Within the profession, laughing at the patient cements the community. If you and I, Doctor, laugh at the same things, we are comrades. We are insiders, with all the privileges accruing to such a status and all the primitive protections it offers. If we laugh at patients, our deepest selves believe that we will not become patients.

Significantly, patients feel free to publish their comic views of physicians (though after he blasted doctors in *The Doctor's Dilemma*, Shaw felt that he had better stay healthy). Physicians, in contrast, tend to laugh behind rubber-gloved hands. It would not be seemly for those to whom we entrust our tortured bodies and psyches to have fun at our (considerable) expense. Patients do not allow physicians that degree of humanness.

There are exceptions, of course. The great physician-writer Rabelais mocked patients, but he mocked everyone in a general belief that to provoke laughter was to encourage health. In our own time, the pseudonymous Shamel Shem, author of *The House of God*, had residents all over the country roaring at his hilarious, if morally superior, portraits of the poor slobs on whom the house staff of an urban medical center practiced their emerging skills. Some people must have felt that

Shem let the side down by showing the public that their doctors found them funny. He broke ranks in another way too. He laughed at his colleagues, a comparatively rare form of professional comedy. Winston Churchill's Rule 6 remains a hard precept to follow for medical comics.

In addition to satiric survival, comedy has even more sustaining roles to play in medicine. But here it is necessary to leave the world of concrete examples for the moment and adduce a little theory.

As every educated person knows, Aristotle believed that when we view a tragedy of a certain proportion, we experience a sensation of being purged of the feelings of terror and pity that the tragedy arouses. Good son of a physician that he was, Aristotle termed the sensation "catharsis." Living honestly through a tragedy—modern psychologists might call it "working through"—we feel cleansed. Terror, pity, and grief are washed through us, and we feel relieved even exhilarated.

Comedy is also cathartic. We have all experienced it as such. The thoroughgoing laugh that we call, significantly, a belly laugh makes us feel oddly better afterwards. At such times, our minds and bodies seem to merge into one enormous, enjoyable reaction. We not only think something is funny; we not only feel something is funny; we know it with our entire selves. That sort of wholeness may be healing. At least we believe it in a folksy way to be so. The millions of readers of the *Reader's Digest* column, "Laughter, the Best Medicine," have casually affirmed laughter's healthful powers over many years. François Rabelais, to whom I alluded earlier, also believed that when he made his patient-readers laugh, he was participating in their cure. And Norman Cousins in his *Anatomy of an Illness* asserted that he had deliberately and successfully sought to use comedy as therapy for his ankylosing spondylitis, a claim that is currently being investigated scientifically, I understand, with early, positive results. Playwrights allude to the cathartic effects of comedy when they speak of inserting a light scene into the middle of a serious drama as "comic relief." That reaction, relief, is also a cause of laughter, according to certain theorists. For instance, Herbert Spencer and, later, Freud, based their theories of laughter on the nineteenth-century hydraulic model in science. In all these cases, laughter becomes as much physical as mental. Osler would understand that. His equanimity consisted in part of imperturbability, which he saw as a bodily endowment.

We sometimes seek this physical relief involuntarily in the midst of tense situations. We laugh when we are nervous. We laugh when we are embarrassed, and our bodies relax. Adults as well as children get giggling "fits." It is our great good fortune that our bodies and minds allow us this relief even in times of great sorrow.

One marvelous illustration of such laughter occurred on the old *Mary Tyler Moore* television comedy during the episode on the death of Chuckles the Clown. It is so hilarious, yet warm-hearted, an instance of comedy in the midst of suffering that it ought to be included in every medical school's teaching about dying, death, and grief. The story is an example of the relief theory of comedy and also the incongruity theory as developed by Kant, Schopenhauer, and dozens of successors. The latter theory hold—to cite the most famous illustration—that we laugh at a pompous, formally dressed man who slips on a banana peel because the juxtaposition is ridiculously incongruous.

As you will remember, Moore's character, also called Mary, works in the newsroom of a television station. Mary charms us because of her innocent goodness, which is often tested by the tougher journalists around her. One of the other recurring characters is the host of the station's children's show, a man always seen in his persona of Chuckles the Clown. One day Mary walks into the newsroom to learn that Chuckles has just died. She is shocked to see that her colleagues are laughing about it. It seems that Chuckles has been killed in the line of duty. Normally dressed as a clown, he had costumed himself as a giant peanut to march in a large parade down the main streets of Minneapolis. As fate would have it, he strutted his peanutty stuff directly in front of the parade's elephants, one of whom—seeing before his disbelieving eyes the morsel of his life—reached out his eager trunk and stuck poor old Chuckles in his mouth, with the inevitable results. The good Mary berates the laughers. How can they carry on so when the life of a fellow human being has been snuffed out in the most unpredictable fashion? He was a colleague, he was a friend, he was a good clown. The laughers are properly remorseful. Seeing that Mary is quite right, they prepare themselves in soberer fashion for the memorial service.

In the next scene, which takes place at the funeral home, they all sit quietly in rows, listening to the minister eulogize their departed comrade. He gave his life for the children, the minister says. In the last role of his existence, Chuckles became a giant peanut marching down Hennepin Avenue. Suddenly, Mary begins to snicker. She inserts first her finger, then her entire hand, into her mouth to stop the giggles. But she cannot help herself. Her body shakes with largely silent chuckles; occasionally we hear an escaping snort. As the minister comes to the part in the story about the elephant, Mary loses control. Opening her mouth, she roars with deep belly laughs and falls off her chair on the floor. Everyone else is shocked. But Mary and her audience have experienced comic catharsis. We all feel much better. As one of Shaw's characters in *The Doctor's Dilemma* says, "Life does not cease to be funny when people die any more than it ceases to be serious when people laugh." As if in further illustration of Shaw's profoundly human paradox, when Mary's laughter is validated by the minister, she bursts into tears.

Comedy's adherence to medicine is abetted by their mutual scientific base. I am here using "scientific" in a broad sense. In literature, in medicine, in daily life, we are operating scientifically when we use our observational, analytical skills and make generalizations based on them. Comedy's scientific basis requires further explanation. Theorists of comedy have tended to agree that it draws on the mind, whereas tragedy plays to the feelings. The idea is that after viewing a tragedy, you are supposed to feel drained. The assumption is that you have to feel bad before you can feel better. In contrast, comedy distances the observer, thereby disengaging the emotions and freeing the rational, scientific part of our response. Even after a fit of belly laughing, wherein the mind seems temporarily to be submerged, our mentation is often clearer.

In interesting contrast to most dramatists, the German playwright, Bertolt Brecht, worried about play-goers becoming too involved with his characters. He felt that an emotionally engaged audience is an exploited audience, victims of the playwright's values. In order to free their minds to reflect rationally upon the serious ideas he was offering, Brecht used several devices to alienate the audience. He would, for instance, follow the figures in *Mother Courage and Her Children* through war-torn, poverty-stricken, and disease-ridden Europe, then instruct someone to cross the stage bearing a sign that said "next day" or "four hours later." "Oh," says the audience, "this is only a play. We need not suffer so much with these people that we ourselves are inert. We must instead think about what we can do to prevent such suffering in the future." Comedy similarly clears the mind. So does science. They keep us from being overly involved with the human data so that we can make effective generalizations.

Then what about compassion? Is there a danger that the physicians who hone their practice of the comic spirit will simultaneously curtail the compassion that is so exquisitely needed in medicine? A parallel question is, does Osler's advice about equanimity, with his chilly talk of obtuseness and imperturbability, limit the heart too much? The nature and training of the humane medical sensibility are subjects too large for this lecture, but, in passing, I want to offer one observation on compassion. Perhaps compassion is not a feeling, but a feeling added to a thought. Might not the formula for compassion be one part vulnerability to the suffering of others plus one part understanding? To the extent that comedy allows doctors to disentangle their feelings from their cognition and frees them to act on behalf of patients, it can serve compassionate ends.

If comedy is akin to science, it is also akin to religion. Considered by some thinkers to be science's opposite, religion is seen in this context to be its completion. I am not now speaking of comedy as it operated in my earliest definitions. Some comedy is satire induced by feelings of superiority, as I have said. Whether through physiological relief or perceptions of incongruity, comedy may also be a mode that stimulates catharsis. But when I speak of comedy's spiritual components, I mean comedy as a point of view that transcends all of that. It transcends even tragedy.

Many thinkers, two poets among them, have led me roundabout to this conclusion. As a child, you probably read William Blake's poems. His *Songs of Innocence*, especially, are widely thought to be pleasant entertainment for children. One of them depicts a brief dialogue between the poet and a newborn child.

Entitled "Infant Joy," it is a simple, direct celebration of new life,

> Pretty joy!
> Sweet joy but two days old.
> Sweet joy I call thee:
> Thou dost smile.
> I sing the while
> Sweet joy befall thee.

But Blake also wrote *Songs of Experience*, some of which are parallels to the "Innocence" poems. The newborn appears again as "Infant Sorrow." In the language of experience, the babe comes,

> Into the dangerous world . . .
> Helpless, naked, piping loud:
> Like a fiend hid in a cloud.

Blake seems to be saying that if we believe that life is jolly, pretty, and quaint, we are looking through eyes of Eden-like innocence. Give us a little experience of the world, and we know joy and sorrow, good and evil. There is not anyone sitting here today who has not lived deeply in the arena of experience.

But this dichotomy is not the end of Blake's vision. Scarcely anyone reads his later poems some of which are obscure, prophetic pieces. Taken together, they reveal what certain readers have called a "higher innocence," a state wherein tragedy is fully acknowledged but as only a penultimate state. Ultimately, if we use our imagination, which is, for Blake, a higher mental functioning than mere reason, we go on to a second innocence. We become fully human, which is tantamount to divine. In that state, we see through all of life's ills to a kind of wise serenity. Here, at last, is my point: Blake's higher innocence is comedy.

The poet Friedrich Schiller gives us another perspective on this kind of comedy. In his essay *On Simple and Sentimental Poetry* he notes comedy's penchant for promoting lucidity of mind. He adds that, through comedy, we view life's absurdities with a smile rather than anger or tears. And he concludes that

> if tragedy sets out from a more exalted place . . . comedy aims at a more important end; and if this end could be actually attained it would make all tragedy not only unnecessary, but impossible.

It is a short step from Schiller to the American mystic Thomas Kelly, who said that finally there is nothing to be afraid of anywhere.

It seems clear to me that people who manifest the most equanimity operate largely in this comic mode. But, for doctors, the perspective will nonetheless present problems since the point of view of the seriously ill patient will almost always be tragic, especially in the early stages of the illness.

By classical—i.e. Greek—definition, tragedy ends death. It is concerned with an important individual, whom it isolates from the community while he or she works out ultimate meanings in relatively ponderous rhythms. In just these ways does the seriously ill patient view matters tragically. For that patient the self is enormous and all-consuming. The patient's problem looms so large as to dominate almost entirely the lens used for looking at the world. The patient's space is constricted, and life becomes comparatively static. He sits in bed and waits. Possible death is the event against which to measure all other experiences.

Enter the busy doctor, who is visiting the patient as one among many on hospital rounds, and will depart in a few minutes. The doctor uses several lenses, whatever is required, to look at many different patients. He or she represents continuity, connectedness with others, *staying on*. The word "rounds" itself suggests as much. Classical comedy had the same purposes. In comedy, people survived. They were seen in relationship to the mundane community. Permanence through renewal was assumed, and in fact Greek comedy arose out of the fertility rites used by primitive peoples to celebrate the returning seasons.

The doctor moves on to other patients. The doctor does not die. Meanwhile, the patient is digging deeper and deeper into a tragic story. Herein lies a clue to one of medicine's frequently cited communication problems. It is easy to see that the doctor's and patient's points of view, the comic and the tragic, are not congruent. They intersect only briefly. It may help to remember that comedy and tragedy have traditionally been considered to be different not in substance, but in perspective. As someone once put it, "Comedy is tragedy— plus time."

What a fine accompaniment is comedy for physicians on their rounds of illness, suffering, and death! They are fools who do not respect these tragedies, and brutes who do not give them their proper dignity. Yet in spite of them, life is connected to life. Other patients wait. Other physicians will follow. Best of all, doctors have special access to the deeply human laughter that allows them to forgive the world, as Osler suggested, for its foibles and uncertainties, and justly to forgive themselves.

Bibliographical Note

I have chosen not to weight this paper down with scholarly attachments. Oslerians may wish to know, however, that the most efficient way to begin a study of comedy is probably through *The Philosophy of Laughter and Humor,* edited by John Morreall for the State University of New York Press in 1987. Morreall introduces selections from both traditional and contemporary theorists. More specifically literary thinkers can be found in *The Comic in Theory and Practice,* edited by

John J. Enck, Elizabeth T. Forter, and Alvin Whitney, and published in 1960 by Appleton-Century-Crofts.

The 'Open Arms' Reviving: Can We Rekindle the Osler Flame? *

John Nicholas Walton (Lord Walton of Detchant)

Robert P. Hudson, former Chairman, Department of the History and Philosophy of Medicine, The University of Kansas noted,

It is a congenial conjunction of fates that brings Oslerians a McGovern Lecturer who shares many of the qualities of the man for whom our Society is named. Such was distinctly the case when Sir John Walton was invited to Birmingham, Alabama, in April 1989 to ask if the Osler flame could be rekindled.

Although I was privileged to share only two days with Sir John, I did not hesitate to accept the honor of writing this short preface to his lecture. He is the sort of man, who, if he chooses, reveals much of himself in a short time. I enjoyed him at the table as a raconteur whose conversation sparkled with erudition and wit, as it played out in a sort of point-counterpoint with his charming wife, Lady Betty. In a somewhat more formal setting I found him to be a riveting public speaker. I was privileged to watch him in the role of clinical consultant, and was reminded what a work of art and science can be forged from a clinical history and neurological examination in the hands of a master. In that same episode I saw in him a supremely humane physician as he explained to the patient that even though medicine could do nothing for her basic disease, it could do much for her and her illness.

Lord Walton's vita came to me as a document of twenty-one pages, sans an ounce of fat. In my allotted space I must, perforce, omit many achievements that would stand out in an average biography. Indeed, it might have been easier to list the honors his accomplishments should have, but did not bring him. He centered his for-

*Delivered 26 April 1989 at the Nineteenth Annual Meeting of the American Osler Society, Birmingham, Alabama.

mal higher education at the University of Durham (M.B., B.S. 1945; M.D. 1952). His principal academic, administrative and clinical focus was at Newcastle upon Tyne where he rose to be Professor of Neurology (1968-1983) and became Dean of Medicine (1971-1981). From 1983 to 1989 he served as Warden, Green College, Oxford.

He has served as editor or board member of seven neurological journals, was Chairman of the Education Committee and later President of the General Medical Council, President of the British Medical Association (1980-1982), President of the Association of British Neurologists, and President of the Royal Society Medicine from 1984-1986. He was made Knight Bachelor in 1979. Shortly following his Osler Society address, Her Majesty the Queen conferred a life peerage on John Walton in her Birthday Honours List in June 1989. He has now taken his seat in House of Lords and has been gazetted as Baron Walton of Detchant in the County of Northumberland.

Underpinning this remarkable public and peer recognition has been a prodigious literary cascade. He has authored or edited twelve books, more than thirty chapters in books, and some 185 papers, and still they come.

Oslerians worldwide rejoiced over the efforts of those who led and contributed to the preservation of Osler's Oxford residence, 13 Norham Gardens. Lord and Lady Walton occupied this historic home for many years.

However trite it may seem, I must begin by saying that it is a singular privilege to have been invited by the Society of which I am now deeply honoured to be an honorary member to give this annual lecture named after that most distinguished physician, founder member and past-President of this Society, Dr. Jack McGovern.

My own interest in medical history was first fuelled in my student days in the medical school of King's College, Newcastle, of the University of Durham, when early in the course I was introduced by an enthusiastic teacher to Osler's writings. Despite the constraints of wartime and of the student purse, I explored and searched whenever I could the bookshops of Tyneside; and when my colleagues sent me as a delegate to London meetings of the British Medical Students' Association, I scrutinised equally avidly those of Gower Street and the Charing Cross Road (especially the second-hand sections of H. K. Lewis and of Foyles) to collect whatever I could of Osler's writings. Having devoured Cushing's *Life of Sir William Osler*,[1] which I believe to be one of the greatest; if not the greatest, medical biography ever written, I moved on to Fulton's *Life of Cushing*[2] and many other biographies and autobiographies, both serious and popular, from pens as varied as those of Howard Haggard, Benjamin Ward Richardson, Johannes Freund, Oliver St. John Gogarty, Arturo Castiglioni, and many more. I was, however, most affected by Osler's *Aequanimitas and Other Essays*,[3] including particularly that on "The student life"[4] which, despite the rather quaint, even archaic language, had a lasting impression upon me, engendering a reverence for Osler and his works which has lasted throughout my professional life. To find myself now, as Warden of Green College, responsible for the maintenance and upkeep of 'The Open Arms' at 13 Norham Gardens, where my wife Betty and I will soon take up residence, is a privilege and responsibility which I treasure greatly. As you are aware, we established some three years ago, with the support and active participation of this Society and of the Osler Club of London, the Friends of 13 Norham Gardens to help me and my colleagues in Green College to fulfill that task.

And before medical and scientific writing on topics like muscular dystrophy and neurological medicine became an abiding interest of mine and occupied most of my writing hours, I first put pen to paper for a medical student journal in 1944 and 1945 in two articles, the first on "Osler: a Great Physician" and the second on "Thomas Sydenham: the English Hippocrates." And later I was privileged in 1969 to deliver the Annual Osler Lecture to the Canadian Medical Association in Halifax, Nova Scotia. And when I handed over the Presidency of the British Medical Association (BMA) at its 150th anniversary meeting in 1982 to His Royal Highness the Prince of Wales, Stephen Lock, the editor of the *British Medical Journal*, independently invited myself and the other BMA chief officers to write articles on "The medical book I would most like to have written;" our articles were published in the *Journal* on 5 July, Vol. 2, 1982. I chose unhesitatingly Cushing's *Life of Osler* [5] which, as I said at the time, gave a superb pen picture of the master, perhaps a trifle dated in its prose but nevertheless a truly great biography. How interesting is it to note that without any collusion Mr. Tony Grabham (now Sir Anthony), then chairman of the BMA Council, chose *Aequanimitas*[6] for its lasting kindly message, as did Mr. David Bolt,[7] Chairman of the Central Committee for Hospital Medical Services, who remarked that his ambition was perhaps less to have written this book than to be the kind of man who could have written it.

13 Norham Gardens: 'The Open Arms'

In his will, Sir William left his house to his wife, expressing the desire that on her death (or earlier if she so wished) the house be given to Christ Church College, of which he was a professorial fellow, "as the residence of the Regius Professor of Medicine." Sir William died in 1919. Lady Osler, who died in 1928, followed in her will Sir William's wishes, and left the house to the Dean and Chapter of Christ Church to be "assigned by them as an official residence of the Regius Professor of Medicine in the University of Oxford for the time being, or to be otherwise applied by the said Dean and Chapter towards the endowment of the chair . . . in such manner as they might think fit." The contents of the house were left by Lady Osler to her brother, Mr. E.H.R. Revere, who in turn conveyed much of the furniture to Christ Church, and Mrs. Susan Chapin (Lady Osler's sister) attended to the arrangements. Some items of furniture were also offered to other members of the Revere family. But some of it which was still serviceable remained in 13 Norham Gardens. Sir Farquhar Buzzard on being appointed Regius Professor of Medicine in 1929 did not wish to occupy the house, and it was let by Christ Church successively to two tenants, first Miss H. L. Hurlston and later a Miss Fairburn. And for a time during the Second World War the house was used to house part of the Mathematical Institute and as a hostel for the Society of Home Students which later became St. Anne's College. In 1953 Christ Church conveyed the property to the University to be held on trust, the trust being expressed in the same terms as in Lady Osler's will, and the University then became the Osler Trustees. Sir George and Lady Pickering took over the tenancy when Sir George came to Oxford to become Regius Professor of Medicine in 1956 and remained there until 1968, when he was succeeded by Sir Richard Doll who, with Lady Doll, lived there until 1979. The new Regius Professor of Medicine, Henry Harris, then decided that he did not wish to take over the lease when appointed in 1979, and for some time the house remained vacant; some furniture was then stored and some was transferred to the country home of the Regius Professor in the almshouses at Ewelme. Some was distributed to other parts of the world including, for example, one of Osler's desks which went to the Osler Library at McGill University in Montreal. Another desk had previously been given to Dr. Palmer Howard in Iowa and other items of furniture had been handed down through the Revere family to Miss Revere of Boston, who still lives on Beacon Hill.

In 1982 the University decided that as the house had been vacant for some time, it should "otherwise apply it towards the endowment of the Regius Professorship"; it therefore leased the house to Green College for twenty-one years from 1 August 1982, on condition that a quarter of the gross income received by the college from lettings of apartments and office accommodation therein would be paid to the Osler Trust, to bear part of the cost of the Regius Professor's stipend. Provision was made in the agreement that an apartment suitable for occupancy by a future Regius Professor of Medicine would be made available. At the same time, it was agreed that the University Newcomers Club could occupy part of the premises on a sub-lease.

It is fascinating now to note the scale of the accommodation available in 13 Norham Gardens in 1929 just after Lady Osler's death. Apart from the large garden, garage, greenhouse and conservatory, there was a huge basement area with a kitchen, scullery, servants' hall, larder, wine cellar and other storage space, while on the ground floor, in addition to a very large hall, there were four reception rooms and a water closet (WC). The first floor (second in American terminology) had a boudoir, seven bedrooms, a dressing room, two bathrooms, two WCs and a housemaid's pantry, while on the second floor (or third, if you wish) were four bedrooms, a linen room, boxroom, sewing room, two bathrooms and again two WCs. When Green College took over the lease, funds were raised from Osler admirers both in the UK and overseas to carry out a programme of conversion through which four small apartments were created in the north end of the building, to be occupied by married students of the college. Three ground floor rooms and an area of the basement were allocated to the Newcomers Club, leaving the large entrance hall, the Osler library and the large adjacent office (formerly Lady Osler's drawing room) to be available for letting, as well as the spacious self-contained Regius Professor's apartment. From 1982 to 1989 that apartment was occupied by a Senior Visiting Research Fellow of Green College, Dr. Philippe Shubik, and he also rented the library and office in order to pursue his work in the field of toxicology and carcinogenesis.

Furniture and Memorabilia. As I have mentioned, one of Osler's desks from 13 Norham Gardens is now in the Osler Library at McGill and another is with Dr. Palmer Howard of Iowa. Some tables from the library remain in 13 Norham Gardens, as do the panelled walls and bookshelves, but some of the original chairs are now in the Regius Professor's apartment at Ewelme. However, the original terrace furniture is still available on the terrace at 13 Norham Gardens and was generously revarnished by Dr. and Mrs. Shubik.

The Acland Triptych. In about 1871, Sir Henry Acland, then Regius Professor of Medicine, commissioned Julian Drummond to make copies of portraits of Linacre, Sydenham and Harvey from the Royal College of Physicians and these were mounted in a triple frame and hung over the fireplace in Sir Henry Acland's library at 39 Broad Street, where the new Bodleian Library in Oxford now stands. When Osler paid his first visit to Oxford in 1894 to attend a meeting of the British Association for the Advancement of Science, he lunched with Sir Henry and was much attracted by the triptych. Mrs. Osler asked Sir Henry if she could have it copied to give to William for a birthday present; the copy went first to the Oslers' home in Baltimore, later being taken to Norham Gardens and installed in the library when Sir William became Regius Professor in 1907. When Sir Farquhar Buzzard in 1929 decided that he did not intend to live there, Dr. William W. Francis, then the Osler Librarian, with the permission of Lady Osler's executors, removed the portraits of Linacre, Harvey and Sydenham from their frames in the panelled library at 'The Open Arms' and took them to McGill where they now hang in a corner of the Osler Room in the McIntyre Building. The three frames remained empty until December 1986 when Dr. Alastair Robb-Smith, an Honorary Member of this Society and President of the Friends of 13 Norham Gardens, generously presented to the Osler Trustees (the University and Green College acting on their behalf) photographic facsimiles prepared by Mr. David Dickinson of the original portraits; these have been mounted into frames in the overmantel by Mr. Frank Samuels, so that the library fireplace in 13 Norham Gardens appears as it did in the illustration in Cushing's *Life of Osler*.[1] Again through the energy and interest of Dr. Robb-Smith, the portrait of Sir Thomas Browne, author of *Religio medici*,[8] one of Osler's favourite works, which used to hang in the library of 13 Norham Gardens but which is now in Pembroke College, has been copied and suitably framed and now hangs in the study.

Other Memorabilia. While Osler's own collection of medical books and incunabula went, of course, to McGill University to establish the Osler Library, Green College is fortunate in having retained many of Osler's own publications including, for example, a first edition of his *System of Medicine* of 1910,[9] two copies of the *Bibliotheca Osleriana* of 1929,[10] and other notable works. We have also received from Mr. E. V. Quinn, former librarian of Balliol, many additional books and papers which he had purchased and which had previously been the property of Miss Mabel FitzGerald, a physiologist and friend of the Oslers who, being a woman, was not able to graduate in her youth from Oxford University but who was finally awarded an honorary MA at the age of one-hundred. These are now housed in the Fellows' Room of Green College, but are the property of the Friends and will be restored to the library of 13 Norham Gardens as the process of refurbishment continues. Some small items of china belonging to Sir William and Lady Osler are still in the library; a set of etchings by Revere Osler was generously donated by Dr. George Harrell, a head of Osler by Doris Appel by Dr. John P. McGovern; a plaque commemorating the contributions of Lady Osler was given by Jefferson Medical College, Philadelphia, and another commemorating Osler's membership of the American Neurological Association by that association. Books have also been donated by Dr. Alec Cooke, Dr. Palmer Howard and Dr. Charles Roland, among others, while Dr. Glenn Knotts of Houston has given the Abram Belskie Medal of Osler created in 1972 to commemorate the foundation of the American Osler Society in Houston, Texas, in 1969. We were also amused to receive from Dr. W. M. Ramsden a silver cigarette case given by Sir William to his uncle, Dr. Walter Ramsden, with a card inscribed in Osler's handwriting saying: "Smoke and think of your good friend, William Osler!" And in May 1984 we received from Professor Michael Brain, son of the late Lord Brain, the D. Sc. gown worn by Sir William Osler when he received that honorary degree from Oxford University in 1904, when the British Medical Association held its annual meeting there. That gown was later given by Lady Osler to Dr. Walter Morley Fletcher, first Secretary of the Medical Research Council, who in turn passed it on to his son, Charles Fletcher; he suggested to Lord Brain that the gown should be converted into a Doctor of Medicine (DM) gown and given to the Royal College of Physicians of London, to be worn by College lecturers who hold an Oxford DM. However, the College already possessed such a gown and Sir Russell Brain, as he then was, said that he would prefer to give it, after conversion at his expense, to his son Michael, then a medical student, if and when he became an Oxford DM. In 1984

Michael Brain (now Professor of Medicine at McMaster University) decided to donate the gown to Green College for display in 13 Norham Gardens, so that it would be available for wear by any future Regius Professor of Medicine or by any Warden of Green College holding a DM of Oxford. The gown is now suitably displayed in the hall. And I am sure that many members of the audience will have read with interest Michael Brain's account of his father's contacts with Osler in Oxford in 1919 published in the *British Medical Journal* on 9 January 1988.[11]

Repairs, Restoration and Visitors. I and the fellows and members of Green College are very conscious of the burden of responsibility that we have accepted in taking over the lease of 'The Open Arms.' While the appeal of the early 1980s launched by my predecessor, Sir Richard Doll, raised substantial funds to assist in converting the house, it became clear soon after Green College took over the lease that as this was on a full repair and maintenance basis, the college faced a major financial burden in simply maintaining its exterior fabric. In 1984 we learned that at least £50,000 would be required to carry out such a programme over a five- to six-year-period. Hence in 1984 an appeal was launched to Osler admirers the world over, including members of the nineteen Osler societies then in existence. We are very grateful to all of those, many present today, who have given substantial donations or have agreed to contribute by deed of covenant to assist us in fulfilling the task. I would like to pay a very warm tribute to the Osler Societies the world over which have supported us, including this Society, the Osler Club of London, and the Japanese Osler Society vigorously led by Dr. Hinohara. Much invaluable support has also come from individuals in the UK but most notable have been the very generous contributions made by Dr. Jack McGovern in whose honour I am speaking today and who is now the Honorary Life President of the Friends. I must also say a very special thank you to Dr. Jeremiah Barondess and to his many colleagues in this Society for the successful approaches they made to colleagues and institutions in the United States, and to Dr. William Spaulding for his noble efforts in raising money for the Friends in Canada. A full list of contributions, both individual and institutional, was given in the *13 Norham Gardens Newsletter* No. 4, and is also displayed in the hallway at 13 Norham Gardens. These donations will make it possible for us now to complete this year the final programme of repairs involving much replacement of decaying stonework on the roof and gable ends of the building, on the entrance steps, on the terrace and above the bay windows, as well as repairs to the lead and slatework on the roof, pointing and restoration of brickwork and replacement of decaying wood.

Even during this programme of repair and refurbishment, it has been our great pleasure to welcome notable visitors from many countries who have come to see the Osler shrine. Among them have been physicians from the Netherlands, from Japan, from the Danish Osler Society, from the Osler Club of London, an international group who came on the *Osler Revisited* conference organised by Nicholas Dewey, a group of US physicians serving in Germany led by Bill Smith, a conference of UK postgraduate deans, Dr. and Mrs. R. McConnell of Liverpool, and many members of this Society including Jerry Barondess, Jim Warren, Nicholas Davies, Robert Kimbrough, Jim Reuler and David Mumford, and David Clarke (a Montreal student who was President of the McGill University Osler Society).

The Future. And what of the future? It is the intention of the Friends of 13 Norham Gardens during the next few years not only to see that Osler's former home is restored to a little approaching its former glory, but also to try to rekindle the Osler flame of international friendship between doctors, medical students and their families, and to make 'The Open Arms' a place which will be regarded by Osler's many disciples as being a fitting tribute to his memory and as helping to maintain the counsels and ideals which made him so famous. The University Newcomers Club, with its active programme for the wives and families of visitors to Oxford from other parts of the UK and from all over the world, is in one sense fulfilling this ideal. However, I am now happy to confirm that as the present Regius Professor does not wish to occupy the apartment at 13 Norham Gardens, the officers of Green College have invited my wife and myself to take over the lease of the apartment on relinquishing the Wardenship of Green College this year; this we have gladly agreed to do. I have now raised the funds necessary to cover the costs of rental of the downstairs offices; and I intend to restore as best I can the library and office as a proper memorial to Osler, and to pursue a number of research projects in neurology and in the history of medicine from this exciting base.

Rekindling the Osler Flame

But rekindling the Osler flame does not only mean refurbishing his former Oxford home. At a time in medicine when resource constraints have beset medical care, medical education and medical research throughout the world, all of us working in these fields should surely do what we can, despite these difficulties, to recall and to instill in those whom we teach and to whom we offer our example in clinical practice the principles so clearly enunciated by Sir William in his writings. How interesting it is to speculate upon what might have happened had Osler taken the alternative path upon which he had set his heart when he first came to London in September 1872 at the age of 23. As a student, he was much impressed by R. Palmer Howard, Professor of Medicine at McGill in 1870-1872, and it was Howard's ambition that William should train in ophthalmology with the ultimate objective of joining the teaching staff of McGill and of Montreal General Hospital. When Canon Osler and William's brothers managed to raise the money needed to support him in his proposed programme of two years in the UK, he first found himself working in the Physiology Laboratory of University College, London, with John Burdon Sanderson. Nevertheless he was determined to emulate, if he could, William Bowman, England's best-known and most talented ophthalmologist. It was Bowman's advice that Osler should begin by working in physiology. While he was doing so the disturbing news came to him from Palmer Howard that a more senior candidate for the post of ophthalmologist in Montreal, Frank Buller, had emerged. It also turned out that Buller was an applicant for the house surgeon appointment at Moorfields upon which young William had set his heart. In the event, as Buller was appointed, Osler decided not to train in ophthalmology but, following in Howard's footsteps, to cultivate the whole field of medicine as it had never been cultivated before.

It is, of course, easy to pick out from Osler's writings many aphorisms as valid today as they were in his time. Neurologists like myself might perhaps question his comment that "Probability is the rule of life, especially under the skin. Never make a positive diagnosis." But in these days of AIDS and of the growing problem of alcoholism in our society, one can only reflect upon his apposite dictum: "Who serves the gods dies young—Venus, Bacchus, and Vulcan send in no bills in the seventh decade." He repeated similar advice in a letter on "Rules for a sensible young fellow," written to A. L. Smith on 20 March 1907, recently resurrected by Giles Bullard in the 1986 Balliol Record and brought to my attention by Nicholas Dewey. His comment to the effect that "Common sense nerve fibres are seldom medullated before forty—they are never even seen with the microscope before twenty" should perhaps be assessed along with the saying of Oliver Wendell Holmes the elder, whom he much admired, who wrote that "Science is a first-rate piece of furniture for a man's upper storey if he has common sense on the ground floor." I always enjoyed, too, his wry comment on one of the medical fashions of his age when he said that "the mental kidney more often than the abdominal is the one that floats." And how could one forget that "although one swallow does not make a summer, one tophus makes gout and one crescent malaria."

What a wonderful teacher Osler must have been. When one reads again his essay on "Teacher and student," in which he stressed the importance of acquiring a significant core of knowledge, based on the appreciation of principles rather than on the cramming of fact, he emphasised system and method, pointing out a lesson which all too many medical students found it difficult to learn, namely the importance of an orderly arrangement of one's work and the organisation of one's time. While the practice of medicine is indubitably an art, it must be firmly based upon science and scientific reasoning. How surprised I was, having played a major part in writing the General Medical Council's (GMC) Recommendations on Basic Medical Education in 1980, to turn back to Osler and to find that some of what I had fondly imagined might be personal gems were not at all new. Thus in relation to "Thoroughness" he confirmed that it was necessary to acquire a full and deep acquaintance of chemistry, anatomy and physiology and of the great principles based upon them. Students must also become familiar with methods by which knowledge is advanced (i.e. research) and must acquire such a knowledge of diseases and of life emergencies and of the means for their alleviation that they may become safe and trustworthy guides for their fellow men. Only through such an approach did he believe that the sloughs of charlatanism could be avoided. But he also roundly condemned cocksureness of opinion leading to a lively conceit in one's personal powers and stressed the vital importance of humility. I have long shared his admiration for Cowper, who said: "Knowledge and wisdom, far from being one, have oft times no connection. Knowledge dwells in heads replete with thoughts of other men, wisdom in minds attentive to their own. Knowledge is proud that he has learned so much, wisdom is humble that he knows no more." At the end of the day, as you all know, Osler saw as fundamental that master word in medicine which he suggested looms large in meaning. He regarded it, and I quote, as "the open sesame to every portal, the great equaliser in the world, the true philosopher's stone;" he thought that it would make the stupid man bright, the bright man brilliant and the brilliant student steady.[12] And he continued,

> With it all things are possible and without it all study is vanity and vexation. To the youth it brings hope, to the middle-aged confidence, to the aged repose. It has been directly responsible for all advances in medicine during the past 25 centuries. Laying hold upon it, Hippocrates made observation and science the warp and woof of our art. Galen so read its meaning that 15 centuries stopped thinking and slept until awakened by Vesalius, the very incarnation of the master word. Harvey gave impulse with its inspiration to a larger circulation than he recognised, Hunter sounded all its heights and depths and stands out in our history as one of the great examples of its virtue. With it, Virchow smote the rock and the waters of progress gushed out, while in the hands of Pasteur it proved a very talisman to open to us a new heaven in medicine and a new earth in surgery.

As you are all well aware, the master word was "work."

Osler the Philosopher

Not only, of course, was Osler a great physician and teacher, but it was clear from all that he wrote that he loved his profession and served it to the end of his days. The guild of doctors was one he regarded as being of noble ancestry, demonstrating solidarity without insularity, and a progressive character allowing the advance of knowledge and developments in medical science and in patient care, coupled with the all-pervasive benevolence and human understanding so fundamental to its practice. Among the sins which he saw in some colleagues were those of excessive nationalism, unalloyed provincialism and parochialism. When I reread his comments on "Chauvinism in Medicine,"[13] I was reminded of the invitation which came to me in 1987 from the editor of the Oxford Medical School Gazette inviting me to comment upon the seven deadly sins as applied to medicine. This invitation prompted me to consider how these sins, namely lust, intemperance, ire, avarice, sloth, pride and envy, could be interpreted in a medical setting, and of course I concluded that all might at times be relevant, even if their respective importance in relation to medical practice may differ from the way that each is regarded by society as a whole.

Wearing one of my other hats as, until recently, President of the General Medical Council, I confess that if one believed the salacious and sensational commentaries of the tabloid press upon the proceedings of its Conduct Committee, some doctors, driven by *lust*, appear to indulge in incredible, even unmentionable, sexual activities with patients of the opposite sex. But, in fact, the proportion of cases involving sexual misdemeanour is small in comparison with the whole (three out of the fifty-three cases handled by the committee last year)—a tiny problem when compared with the twenty-four doctors accused of serious neglect or disregard of their professional responsibilities to patients (also relatively few when derived from about 100,000 practising doctors in the UK).

Intemperance is, of course, a syndrome not unfamiliar (on occasion) in doctors and we cannot be proud of the fact that until about 1980 the incidence of cirrhosis of the liver was more than three times as great in doctors as in the general population. More recent figures suggest that its incidence in members of the profession is falling, but nevertheless addiction to alcohol or drugs is still by far the commonest cause of reference to the GMC's health procedures. Since 1980 over 150 doctors have been placed under supervision (a few have had their registration suspended) for this cause and about ten doctors a month are now being referred to the National Counselling and Welfare Service for sick doctors.

Of less direct concern to the GMC but nevertheless worrying and troublesome is *ire*. The more I have seen of medicine in forty-two years of clinical practice, the more I have recognised the crucial need for good communication between doctors and patients and the necessity of compassionate and humane management of sick people even when the doctor is weary and even when provoked or irritated by inconsiderate or irrational behaviour (patients, like doctors, sometimes lose their tempers and behave badly). But times out of number, I received letters at the GMC from patients suggesting that doctors had been abominably rude, clumsy, arrogant, thoughtless or just simply unsympathetic, unfeeling or unkind. They said: "I don't want the doctor 'struck off'; please write and ask him (or her) to be nice to people in future"—but that, of course the Council could not do without invoking the full panoply of quasi-legal procedures. *Avarice*, too, falls outside the GMC's statutory powers even though some letters complain about what, prima facie, looks like gross overcharging in private practice. Can we hope that the profession itself, with appropriate procedures at a local level, could satisfy public concern about some such matters?

Sloth, if I interpret the word literally, is I think pretty rare among doctors in clinical practice who are all too often, whether in junior resident posts or even when more senior, overworked and weary. And in family practice, too, the third night call during an epidemic or the stress of coping with an importuning patient in a crowded office can impose almost intolerable strains on a doctor's reserves of patience and understanding. But sick people are often frightened people and the diagnosis of acute meningococcal meningitis or of a perforated appendix in the middle of the night, followed by prompt action, can excuse several unnecessary calls which only an expert could judge with hindsight to have been unnecessary. No, sloth is not usually a problem with doctors—but perhaps the most difficult lesson of all for the young doctor to learn (as I said earlier) is how, in the face of competing demands and responsibilities, to be able to organise his or her time.

And so we are left with *pride* and *envy*. Relevant to medicine? Of course they are. If (with apologies to Rudyard Kipling) pride leads you to rely upon your own skill in diagnosis and management and to be so self-confident as to refuse the legitimate wish of a patient to seek a further (probably confirmatory) opinion, it comes before a fall. If intellectual and professional arrogance cloaks your opinions with an aura (to yourself) of infallibility, if that arrogance leads in turn to an inability or unwillingness to talk to a patient on equal terms with a full and frank discussion of pros and cons, if you are unable or unwilling to admit, on occasion, your uncertainties or even your mistakes, and if pride or envy leads you unjustifiably to criticise or disparage the views or advice given by a professional colleague, these are indeed deadly medical sins. For the days of "doctor's orders" are long past; the doctor-patient relationship is a partnership in which the doctor offers advice, but it is up to the patient to decide whether or not to accept it.

Doctor-Patient Communication

May I now return to the question, so dear to Osler's heart, of communication between doctors and patients? Some of the greatest misunderstandings which arise between doctors and patients and their families occur when this is unsatisfactory. In the medical consultation, the keystone of clinical practice, the interview is the beginning. Interviewing skills can be examined, assessed and taught. It is salutary for a doctor to see a videotape recording of an interview conducted by himself/herself. Even more important is the exposition or discussion in which the doctor must give clear and concise advice but must not strike an authoritarian role. Constraints of time in busy clinics or in overcrowded wards must be admitted. Equally important is the fact that patients often forget, misunderstand, or misinterpret doctors' opinions and advice. Doctors themselves may be at fault by writing extremely complex prescriptions. For this reason, the profession should examine the possibility of producing more written advice to patients about the management of their illnesses. A working party which I chaired at the Nuffield Provincial Hospitals Trust produced a booklet for doctors and medical students ("Talking with Patients") which proved popular. Doctors should always remember that patients may be so distracted by anxiety that they cannot regularly remember what they are told. Sometimes, too, the patient's social and domestic circumstances may inflate or distort the significance of a trivial medical problem. Equally, too, there are patients who either find it impossible, or are unwilling, to comply with doctors' recommendations with regard to treatment.

Communication Between Doctors and Other Doctors and with Other Health Care Professionals

Just as doctor-patient communication is fundamental to good medical practice, communication between doctors in different specialties on the one hand and between doctors and other health care professionals on the other is equally important and often overlooked. The same working party of the Nuffield Provincial Hospitals Trust produced two further booklets highlighting some problems which had emerged as a result of our enquiries into intraprofessional communication. One social worker said to a doctor "I cannot hear what you say while what you are rings so loudly in my ears." But a hospital administrator also said wryly that it was his duty to serve the interests of 200 consultants, 195 of whom owed allegiance only to God and the other 5 did not even accept that limitation. I feel sure, too, that Osler would have felt just as concerned as did Dr. Alec Cooke in the talk he gave to the Oxford meeting of the Osler Club of London a few years ago in which he castigated the profession for its increasing use of acronyms, some of which he found increasingly unintelligible on studying hospital care records. Beginners, he felt sure, would have no difficulty in interpreting the meaning of WR for Wassermann reaction, PM for post-mortem, or D and C for dilatation and curettage. Even more advanced students would usually be quite happy in interpreting GFR, MCHC or DNA but might be compelled to hesitate a little in reading NCT for "not come through" or LSCS for "lower segment Caesarian section." But even honours students, he suggested, might be taken aback by EUAPS for "examination under anaesthetic of post-nasal space," DNSVI for "does not seem very ill," and especially when confronted by the final gem which he had found in a patient's notes as LASNULLLRSR, standing for "local anaesthesia, seventh nerve, upper lid, lower lid and retrobulbar space on the right." Surely, despite the temporal constraints which afflict us all in our clinical practice, we can do better?

Communication with the Media

Many doctors have also learned to their cost that communication with the media needs considerable skill and judgment. Charles Fletcher dealt admirably with this issue in his Rock Carling Lecture in 1972,[14] and quoted with approbation Osler's warning in 1907 that the Delilah of the press may perhaps be courted with satisfaction but sooner or later was sure to play the harlot; it would thus "leave a man shorn of his strength, *viz*. the confidence of his professional brethren." How true that remains today when we all in medicine have been compelled to acknowledge increasing public interest in matters medical. This area, upon which I do not have time to dwell, requires exceptional expertise.

Epilogue

May I finally comment upon some of the fashionable but false antitheses which were so effectively demolished by Sir Douglas Black in his Rock Carling Lecture for 1984?[15] Of his many verbal, philosophical and scientific gems I have time to select very few. When Faraday was asked by one sceptical of the value of science, "What use is electromagnetism?" his response was brief but compelling: "What use is a baby?" he said. All of us in clinical medicine know that there is no antithesis between the scientific and so-called holistic methods or between the scientific and the compassionate and caring, as all doctors, whatever their training and specialty, surely strive to practise whole-patient medicine. I am convinced that the good doctor is just as concerned with disease prevention as with cure. Nevertheless, Black did an invaluable service in stressing that those who feel that management and business skills may be used to buy results in the ever-changing and ever-challenging field of medical research must recognise that 'lavish finance can be impotent in the face of unripe time.' Parkinson in his 'laws of medical research' said much the same thing when indicating that research which does not define precisely a question to be asked, methods of answering it, and a route to be followed may be as fruitless in medicine as is that which goes astray because of deficiencies in clinical knowledge, skills or experience.

As Osler so clearly indicated many years ago, clinical and laboratory science, combined with communication skills, must continue to be partners in our avowed aim of serving to the best of our ability our patients, future patients, knowledge itself and society. These may be truisms but it is upon their full recognition and application in our everyday contact with patients that a proper rekindling of the Osler flame depends.

References

1. Cushing, H. *Life of Sir William Osler*. 2 Vols., Oxford, Clarendon Press, 1925.
2. Fulton, J.F. *Harvey Cushing. A Biography.* Springfield, IL, Charles C. Thomas, 1946.
3. Osler, W. *Aequanimitas. With Other Addresses to Medical Students, Nurses, and Practitioners of Medicine*. 2nd ed., London, H.K. Lewis, 1910.
4. Osler, W. The student life. In: *Aequanimitas, loc cit* #3, p. 413.

5. Walton, J. Medical book I would most like to have written: Life of Osler. *Brit Med J* 150th Anniversary Issue (AI):59, 1982.
6. Grabham, A.H. Medical book I would most like to have written. Aequanimitas: I. *Brit Med J* 150th Anniversary Issue (AI):59, 1982.
7. Bolt, D.E. Medical book I would most like to have written. Aequanimitas: II. *Brit Med J* 150th Anniversary Issue (AI):62, 1982.
8. Browne, T. *Religio medici*. London, Andrew Crooke, 1642.
9. Osler, W. and McCrae, T. *A System of Medicine, by eminent authorities in Great Britain, the United States and the Continent.* 7 Vols. London, Frowde, 1907-1910.
10. Osler, Sir W. *Bibliotheca Osleriana. A Catalogue of Books Illustrating the History of Medicine and Science. . . .* Oxford, Clarendon Press, 1929.
11. Brain, M. Brain and Osler: Collaborations in 1919. *Brit Med J* 296:104-105, 1988.
12. Osler, W. The master-word in medicine. In: *Aequanimitas*, *loc cit* #3, p. 363. (Note: Pagination same as in 1904 edit.)
13. Osler, W. Chauvenism in medicine. In: *Aequanimitas*, *loc cit,* #3, p. 277. (Note: Pagination same as in 1904 edit.)
14. Fletcher, C.M. *Communication in Medicine*. Rock Carling Fellowship Lecture, 1972. London, Nuffield Provincial Hospitals Trust, 1973.
15. Black, D. *An Anthology of False Antitheses.* Rock Carling Fellowship Lecture. London, Nuffield Provincial Hospitals Trust, 1984.

Rx: Hope*

E.A. Vastyan

E.A. Vastyan was the founding chairman, in 1967, of the first Department of Humanities created at a College of Medicine—that at the Pennsylvania State University, Hershey. Under his aegis, the disciplines of ethics, history, literature, philosophy, and religion were incorporated as a required part of the medical curriculum. This was an educational innovation that subsequently spread quite rapidly throughout medical education in America. Instrumental in the adoption of such disciplines in the medical curriculum were such organizations as the Society for Health and Human Values, and the Institute on Human Values in Medicine, on both of which Professor Vastyan served in leadership positions. Through both organizations he also served as a consultant on humanistic studies in medicine at some twenty colleges of medicine; and, as a member of the National Board of Consultants of the National Endowment for the Humanities, at numerous other universities. He lectured and led seminars at many of these schools. For six years he served as an advisory board member of The Robert Wood Johnson Foundation Clinical Scholars Program. Before his appointment at Penn State, he served in an academic chaplaincy at The University of Texas Medical Branch, Galveston, and The Ohio State University, Columbus.

Born in Fairport Harbor, Ohio, Professor Vastyan was awarded the B.A. degree with Honors by Denison University, where he was elected to Phi Beta Kappa; and the B.D. degree *cum laude* by the Episcopal Theological School of Cambridge, Massachusetts. He did graduate study at the University of Southampton, England, the University of Chicago, and Harvard University.

---

*Delivered 8 May 1990 at the Twentieth Annual Meeting of the American Osler Society, Baltimore, Maryland.

In the gloom gold gathers the light about it.

Ezra Pound[1]

Let me open not only with a word of gratitude for the privilege of your invitation, but with a warning as well. In his famous—or as some termed it, infamous—valedictory address at this great institution, which Osler titled "The Fixed Period," he remarked on the "absolute uselessness of men more than 60 years old." That makes the task of my lecture quite carefree, for the men who invited me were fully aware that they had a sexagenarian,—well past 60—in hand. So you must be content with listening to uselessness.

One further warning as well. Oslerians like you all know that not only was he born to a father who was a missionary Anglican priest, but that young Osler himself intended to enter Holy Orders. My warning is this: I, too, am an Anglican priest. My primary vocation, despite the fact that I have been a medical educator for a quarter-century, has been that of ministry. And so, although religion is still often a taboo topic in polite company, my perspective today will be that of religion and of pastoral ministry—and specifically, of the only ministry I know—the Christian ministry.

Although one could make generalizations about hope and spirituality that could be applicable to religion in general, I shall speak admittedly from within the Christian context alone, and hope that the necessary connections to other religious traditions which you may wish to make, can be drawn by inference. I like what Carlyle once said: that he could learn religion only from someone who knew God other than by hearsay. My only experience and knowledge of God—and of hope—are related to my practice of my Christian vocation. I will try rigorously to limit my remarks to what I know from that experience, and hope you will freely draw whatever connections are necessary to connect it with your own spiritual experience, and with your own knowledge and practice of medicine.

One further introductory clarification needs to be made. Let me suggest it with a story. One of my favorite physician-mentors, with whom I frequently made teaching rounds, was not only an excellent clinician, but an excellent teacher. Pithy aphorisms ("pearls" to the students) would fall from him like seed following the sower. Three basic principles, he would tell all medical students, would see them safely through Emergency Room duty: "First, air goes in and out. Second, blood goes round and round. Third, oxygen is good." One day an even wiser colleague corrected him: "Ah, but one more is needed: 'bleeding always stops.'"

So I ask your indulgence for a paper also based on certain very simple presuppositions that I hold, and that I believe apply not only in an emergency room--but in the emergency situation we know as the human condition. My remarks will be those of one who stands frankly and forthrightly on one side of that great, perhaps most basic, divide in humankind: I am a supernaturalist, a theist. I suspect many of you, perhaps even most of you, are naturalists. Further, I believe hope can be understood only by a supernaturalist; certainly hoping behavior is appropriate only for a supernaturalist—one who believes there is meaning and purpose in a spiritual world that is beyond reason, beyond our finite world.

My presuppositions are also simple, also three,

1. God is God, and is in control of every aspect of life—temporal life, and eternal life.
2. We know God as He reveals Himself to us in his Holy Word and Sacraments; and we know him not by inquisitiveness or imagination or inventiveness—but only by obedience.
3. The basic, most fundamental principle of the cosmos is redemptive, not rational. This may be another way of stating the fourth emergency principle above: bleeding always stops.

Another clinical friend has confided to me that when he speaks of a single case in any paper or lecture, he speaks from "my experience." Two patient histories, for him, constitute "a series of cases." Let me now get to the substance of my remarks with the first of "a series of cases" I want to use to frame our consideration of hope.

For some twenty years, one of my standard courses at the College of Medicine at Hershey has been one titled "Dying, Death and Grief." Since most of my students had not yet begun clinical rotations, I assign them to clinical preceptors, with the request that they be assigned to specific patients. Their duties were clearly spelled out: they were to pretend to absolutely no professional expertise, but were to seek the patients' permission to interview them simply as person to person, seeking to understand more deeply what it was like to be seriously ill.

One of our senior faculty members refused to act as preceptor; finally, over a serendipitous lunch one day, told me why. "I'd cooperate," she said, "if you taught it to seniors; but I want those students to learn some real medicine before they see any patients." My counter was that, if such were the case, I would be even more eager to have my turn at bat with the students first. Yet that very afternoon she telephoned me, and asked if I would, in a pastoral capacity, see one of her patients. I'll call him "Brownie."

"I was just with him," she said, "to confide to him that I had exhausted all therapeutic possibilities. That there was no way I knew to delay further the progress of his disease. And," she continued, "he met that with effusive gratitude, almost with joy. I was pretty wiped out by that. Would you visit him?"

I did, and a series of daily visits followed. We not only prayed together; we talked together at length. This was the first time in my experience that I fully realized how important reminiscence can be to a dying patient—a recovering and remembering of the times of life that had been replete with meaning and purpose, as a rich way to launch off into the unknown. Many of his stories were of living through danger during his duty as a bombardier in American Flying Fortresses during World War II.

After about a week, his physician called me again. She had made rather carefully conceived provisions to have Brownie go home, to be with his wife and daughters for his final days. To her surprise, he refused. He wanted to remain in the hospital, and his physician couldn't understand why. Could I shed any light on that, she wondered.

I asked him that afternoon. Instead of responding directly, he began a story: "Our bombing missions would go deep into Germany long before our fighter escorts had the range to go with us. They'd go to the limit of their range, turn back, refuel, and meet us again at their limit on our homeward course. After one particularly rough mission over Berlin, where we had lost many planes, we were limping back to England—badly damaged, with a gunner dead in the tail. Over France, one of our engines had begun to smoke. As I was hunched up there in the bombardier's bubble, an American fighter plane came buzzing past. When he saw how badly we were hurt, he throttled back, pulled almost alongside me in the bubble, and raised his arm in a sign: 'Thumbs up!' I could almost hear him say it. Just as he did it, pow!, an anti-aircraft shell exploded, and his plane disintegrated before my eyes." He paused for a long moment. "That's what I want to do for my family. That's why I want to die here, not at home."

He died a few days later. I wasn't present, but I was later told it had the air of a celebration—with wife, daughters, nurses, residents—singing hymns, and exchanging hugs and kisses and tears.

Experiences like this may be relatively infrequent; they are not unique. Something like it will even be described in medical literature on occasion. Many of you probably saw the moving paper in *The New England Journal of Medicine* a few years ago—by a self-described "successful, hard-driving and competitive" surgeon.[2] Robert M. Mack published a very personal account of what he called the "lessons" he had learned from living with cancer, an adenocarcinoma of the lung. After a successful surgical resection he experienced two years of symptom-free life, until a new growth was discovered in the lung, with metastases to at least three sites of bone. Following a time in which he was "devastated, bewildered and very frightened," he wrote, "I am happier than I have ever been. These are truly among the best days of my life."

He continued: "It became poignantly clear to me . . . that this was a time of real choice. I could sit back and let my disease and my treatment take their course, or I could pause, and look at my life and ask, 'What are my priorities?' . . . One of the really ironic things about the human experience is that many of us have to face pain or injury or even the possibility of death in order to learn the real purpose of being and how best to live a rewarding life."

Dr. Mack's experience was even more eloquently expressed by Senator Paul Tsongas, who titled the memoir of his life with cancer, *Heading Home.*[3] In that book, he wrote,

> The illness made me face up to the fact that I will die someday. It made me think about wanting to look back without regret whenever that happened . . . My illness has forced me to understand that I have true spiritual needs whether I am healthy or unhealthy . . . Now the entire matter of belief is central to me and gives me a truer sense of direction. . . . These changes, or more accurately reinforcements, are a precious gift. The cancer gave them to me. I treasure them.

Such reactions, however, while not rare, are probably not the norm among cancer patients—or among patients with ominous diseases generally. Patients and families, within experience I suspect is common to most of us, are much more often torn by anguish, often tragically crushed by the burden of lethal illness and suffering. Perhaps even more frequently, such patients avoid any outward expression of the effects of their illness, bearing in silence and solitude—and so often in depression and despair—their inner agony.

Yet experiences like those of Brownie, Dr. Mack, Senator Tsongas—are not simply anomalies. I have repeatedly encountered that same affirming joyfulness in patients—and so, too, I suspect, have most nurses and physicians who have been willing to let such patients share their inner lives.[4]

Experiences like these are what I refer to as hoping behavior. What happens in the lives of such people? How shall we understand such reactions to life-threatening illness? How should we respond? Suggestive questions abound,

1. What is it that lies at the root of such behavior?
2. What is the nature of such hope?
3. Can religious concepts—specifically, can Christian concepts—help us understand as well as recognize such hope?
4. What implications would such understanding have for medical care of such patients, when we encounter such behavior?
5. Can we foster such behavior amid the dire circumstances of grief, and suffering, and dying? Should we?

Within the category of medical literature, I've been able to find very little that deals with hope, either explicitly or implicitly. *Index Medicus* has no category for hope. There are, of course, categories that index the psychological and behavioral ramifications of illness, but still very little of Hope or hoping. But a few papers can be found. I have long known, and used, one by Brody, published in *JAMA*[5] And I was surprised last week by a physician-friend who sent me a clipping from the most recent issue of *JAMA* entitled, as was Brody's paper, simply "Hope."[6]

Both are interesting papers. And both assume that hope can be a prescription—an "Rx"—something which can be ordered by the physician and can even be dispensed, to order, by ancillary medical personnel.

Indeed, Buchholz, in that most recent paper, writes with tongue-in-cheek, of hope as a generic product of the pharmacopeia of wise physicians—as "a naturally occurring substance created by an individual's ability to project himself or herself into the future and imagine something better than what exists in the present." He writes, further: "The only limit on maximum dosage is the patient's ability to receive and the professional's ability to administer HOPE at an appropriate rate."

Both papers have valuable suggestions for fostering hope, but I wish to suggest another perspective: that hope is fundamentally a gift to be received—not a behavior or concept or an emotion that can be prescribed.

Further, I want to suggest it is a gift which is received by physician as well, a gift from the patient, a gift which can be fostered, encouraged, wondered at—but which paradoxically, one of the truly great gifts that cannot given, but must be humbly received, by the "care-giver."

I believe it is a myth that we can either "give" or "take away" hope. Moreover, it's a myth that goes with the arrogance of believing the "care-giver" is a spiritually superior person, or in a spiritually superior position. There exists a vast religious experience and literature, ancient as well as modern, which suggest the opposite is almost always the case.

Hope has, however, been relatively neglected, both as a philosophical and theological concept, until relatively recently. Within classical theology, it seems to be the poor third sister among the great theological virtues of faith, love, and hope—often being subsumed in discussions about faith.

Within the past three decades, there has appeared a "Theology of Hope"—usually associated with two German theologians, Jurgen Moltmann and Wolfhart Pannenberg. This has emerged in a strident Marxist form of politics called "Liberation Theology;" what I know of it has not seemed of much use for our purposes in discussing hope in a medical context.

Much more useful to me have been three other Europeans. Two were French philosophers of the World War II era, Gabriel Marcel and Simone Weil, and the third was a transplanted Dutchman, Paul Pruyser, who spent most of his life at the Menninger Clinic as a psychologist of religion.

Marcel produced an important work under the oppression of the Nazi occupation of France, which he called a *Sketch of a Phenomenology and a Metaphysic of Hope*.[7] Simone Weil, during the same period, produced much more modest but, I believe, even more profound, observations in a series of letters and brief essays—the most useful for me being her study of "Affliction and the Love of God."[8] Pruyser both influenced and was influenced by Karl Meninger's own contributions to the study of hope—and is, to the best of my knowledge, the only medically related person to explore the ramifications of Marcel's work.[9-10]

Out of their work, there emerges a strong consensus about some of the basic characteristics of hope. Marcel emphasized a key point: that it is most helpful and useful to talk about the phenomenon as hoping, rather than as hope; to view it always as a verb, rather than a noun. For hoping, he insists, is much more a matter of being than of having, of a process rather than a static entity, of behavior rather than concept.

Hoping, moreover, he sees as a global condition. It affects the whole person, and is directed at what we might term basic purpose or meaning. In this way, it can be clearly differentiated from wishing or desiring—which are usually directed at very specific objects. And to separate hoping from wishing or desiring, understanding its fundamental differences, is key to recognizing it.

The self's involvement in hoping is very different from one's involvement in wishing or desiring. With a wish or desire, I am usually deeply and strongly involved. I develop strong emotional attachment or longing; I engage in obsessive behavior to attain a wish. With hoping, the process is much more quiescent. Hoping always has the nature of humility—of responsiveness, of waiting, really of awaiting.

Another basic, differentiating characteristic of hoping is its communal character. It is different, for instance, from either optimism or pessimism—both of which have an assertive, aggressive element. Both optimist and pessimist tend to say, "If only you could see things as I do." In both there persists a zeal to convert the hearer to my point of view. So, too, to doubt something, or conversely, to assert something, is rooted in the nature of self-assertiveness: *my* point of view should prevail.

Not so with hope. Rooted as it is within calamity or catastrophe, hoping knows deeply a tragic sense of life. And within that knowledge of suffering and anguish, hoping remains always modest. Hoping knows no assertiveness. While it is intimate and private, it is usually shared quietly, without argument, without aggressiveness. It unites rather than divides, even when the auditor (perhaps physician or nurse) does not truly share the hope offered by the hoping person.

It is at this point, Simone Weil observes, that the most significantly spiritual act occurs when hoping appears. She writes, "We possess nothing in this world other than the power to say I. This is what we should yield up to God, and this is what we should destroy." Hoping, for Weil, involves giving up the right to oneself, offering the self as at once a gift-received from God, as a gift-given to God, in an act she terms "de-creation."

These are fundamental characteristics noted by Marcel, Weil, and Pruyser. Let me suggest several more.

I have always found hoping behavior rooted in expectancy. Desiring or wishing, on the contrary, seems almost always rooted in expectation. And the difference between expectancy and expectation is the difference between freedom and bondage.

A strong wish or desire enslaves me very specifically to the object of my longing, my expectation—whether this be romantic love, sexual obsession, or material gratification. Nothing satisfies Mercedes lust but a Mercedes; that poor person can never again drive either happily or safely in a Cadillac. Expectation is always concrete, always pressing, always urgent.

Expectancy is fundamentally different. It is freeing, for it is openness to an open future—a trusting, even eager, waiting for whatever is about to happen. One patient with an ominous cancer once put it this way to me: "I am watching, really eager—to see how God is going to handle this thing." And there's usually an element of joy to the waiting, even to the waiting that is immersed in danger.

For danger is a frequent companion of hope. Hoping appears most characteristically—and some would say, only—under conditions of suffering, of catastrophe, of calamity. C.H. Spurgeon, the great ninteenth century London preacher, put this point succinctly: "Hope is like a star—not to be seen in the sunshine of prosperity, and only to be discovered in the night of adversity."[11] Even more stark is Simone Well: "The dereliction in which God leaves us is his own way of caressing us."

Another element must be strongly emphasized. Hoping never emerges as some decorative aspect of confident living; it is no part of the power of positive thinking, or living. Hoping appears if, and only if, the tragic human condition—of vulnerability, of mortality, of helplessness—is forthrightly faced, accepted—and, finally, both affirmed and celebrated. "Life is the destiny you are bound to refuse," W. H. Auden warns, "until you have consented to die."[12] "Symbolically manifested in the sacrament of Holy Baptism, that dying—giving up one's right to oneself—Auden sees (in common with traditional Christian theology) as the key to hoping behavior, the key to life.

Explore this a bit further with me in our own context in contemporary medicine. Medicine has provided us such awesome relief from suffering, pain, anguish—that we can be easily sidetracked from facing our own personal vulnerability. Indeed, we tend to think it morbid to face either disease or death as an inevitable condition of humankind. And yet, though anesthesia, analgesics, and medical technology have all been remarkable achievements of the past century, the fourth rule of Emergency Room medicine still holds immutable: bleeding always stops. Death comes.[13,14]

Hoping suggests that this basic vulnerability must be recognized, faced, even cherished—in the midst of, in spite of, our technological prowess and human ingenuity. Otherwise our lives are lives of denial, self-deception, and illusion. The prophet Jeremiah expressed this long ago,

> They have healed the wound of my people lightly,
> saying 'Peace, peace,'
> when there is no peace.
>
> (Jeremiah 7:14, NIV)

The Biblical attitude is "always robust . . . there's not the tiniest whine about it . . . there is always a sting and a kick all through the Bible."[15]

The most basic Christian understanding goes even further, suggesting that *living vulnerably* is the only true sharing of the broken human condition, the only true living of hopeful lives, free lives, in this world."[16] Look for instance at the most hallowed teaching of Jesus of Nazareth, in the Beatitudes,

> Blessed are the poor in spirit,
> for theirs is the kingdom of heaven.
> Blessed are those who mourn,
> for they will be comforted.
> Blessed are the meek,
> for they will inherit the earth. . . .
> Blessed are those who are persecuted because of righteousness,
> for theirs is the kingdom of heaven.
> (Matthew 5:3ff, NIV)

This is an insistence that losing is finding, that sharing is possessing, that vulnerability—accepted, affirmed, cherished, lived—is the very key to fulfilled, purposeful life. This was put simply and starkly in a fragment of verse by Puritan divine, Richard Baxter,[17]

> I preached as never sure to preach again,
> And as a dying man, to dying men.

Living hopefully, living vulnerably, in this fashion means one is willing to celebrate the temporary—to accept with a sense of joy all of that which finite, mortal, limited, conditioned, suffering, tragic, broken human life has to offer—as today's life, temporary life, abundant life, all of life. It is this affirmation which lies behind the provision of daily manna to the Israelites wandering in the desert: it was food for today. If you picked enough for tomorrow, it would spoil. If you didn't pick enough, your neighbor had enough to share. So, too, it undergirds the petition in the prayer Jesus taught: Give us this day our daily bread. John Donne emphasized the point eloquently: "We ask *panem quotidianum*, our daily bread, and God never says you should have come yesterday, he never says, you must come again tomorrow, *but today if you will hear his voice*, today he will hear you.[18]

My final point is perhaps but a repeat of all the others—hoping is basically intense concentration on God's point of view. Hoping behavior is a living, daring confidence in God that is so sure, so certain, the hoper would stake his life on it a thousand times. Paul of Tarsus, who lived through shipwrecks, floggings, imprisonments, stonings, could write from his final prison in Rome, before his execution, a letter to the Philippians that is the New Testament's paean to joy—and to hope. To vulnerable, joyful hoping. He concludes: "I have learned to be content whatever the circumstances. I know what it is to be in need, and I know what it is to have plenty . . . I can do everything through him who gives me strength . . . And my God will meet all your needs according to his glorious riches in Christ Jesus." (Philippians 4:10ff, NIV)

Let me conclude with a simple story from personal experience. The wife of a close friend, (I'll call her Hannah) had been rushed to our Emergency Room, and then to intensive care, with severe internal hemorrhaging. Physicians had told her husband that the situation looked bleak. Following a Sunday church service, he asked if I would go with him to visit his wife, and share with them prayers for healing. We went to her bedside in the intensive care unit—where tubes and wires, as usual, stretched everywhere. He greeted her, and began what I thought was superbly understated encouragement: "You are brave, you are superb, you are my love. You're doing well. Hang in there, hang tough." It was a good sermon.

She rasped a response neither of us could understand. He asked her to repeat. She did so in the same words, apparently. Again we couldn't understand. Once more he asked her to repeat; once more with the same result. At the fourth time, she finally opened her eyes and virtually yelled, with feeble strength and failing breath, distinct, individual words, spaced out and clear: "My . . . hand . . . is . . . in . . . the . . . hand . . . of . . . Jesus. "

And it clearly was, for whatever outcome was impending—neither of us could any longer have doubt about that. Hannah survived.

Are there clinical ramifications to these observations? I suggested that I would explore some, but most, I suspect, have already been readily apparent. Yet my major points perhaps should have stark, simple emphasis: There is no technology of hope. There is no technique of hope-giving. There are no professional hope-givers. "Rx: Hope?" No, that's not a prescription a single one of us can write for any human being.

Hope is a gift, a gift of grace to the sufferer, in the midst of suffering, whenever it appears.

It can be a gift from the sufferer, when hope appears, to us—to anyone privileged to be a "care-giver" in the midst of suffering, if we can expectantly accept it.

We can find the gift, and recognize it, accept it—only when we are willing to admit our own vulnerability, our own final helplessness.

And my strong conviction is that we'll find it much more often than we have—if we look for it, if we are willing to find it, if we're willing to accept it, from those who suffer in our presence and under our care. We'll find that hope, and see it in our patients, if we're willing, from time to time, to put aside our expertise and our professionalism—and let heart speak to heart. If we are willing to be free, as one writer put it, "free to be merely man." And, I will add, free to let God be God—the God of hope.

References

1. Pound, Ezra. *The Cantos.* New York, New Directions, 1948.
2. Mack, Robert M. Lessons from Living with Cancer. *N Engl J Med* 311: 1640-1644, 1984.
3. Tsongas, Paul. *Heading Home.* New York, Alfred A. Knopf, 1984.
4. Vastyan, E.A. Spiritual Aspects of the Care of Cancer Patients, *CA-A Cancer J for Clin* 36: 111-114, 1986.
5. Brody, Howard. Hope. *JAMA.* 246: 1411-1412, 1989.
6. Buchholz, William M. A piece of my mind. HOPE. *JAMA* 263:2357-2358, 1990.
7. Marcel, Gabriel. *Homo Viator.* Gloucester, MA, Peter Smith, 1978.
8. Paniches, George A. (Ed.). *The Simone Weil Reader.* New York, David McKay, 1977.
9. Pruyser, Paul W. Phenomenology and Dynamics of Hoping. *J for the Scientific Study of Religion*, Fall, pp. 86-96, 1963.
10. Pruyser, Paul W. Maintaining hope in adversity. *Bull Menninger Clin*, 51: 463-474, 1987.
11. Spurgeon, C.H. *Morning by Morning.* Springdale, PA, Whitaker House, 1984.
12. Auden, W.H. "For The Time Being—A Christmas Oratorio," *The Collected Poetry of W.H. Auden*, New York, Random House, 1945, pp. 407-466.
13. McGill, Arthur C. "Human Suffering and the Passion of Christ." In: Flavian Dougherty, C.P. (Ed.), *The Meaning of Human Suffering*, New York, Human Sciences Press, 1982.
14. McGill, Arthur C. *Suffering: A Test of Theological Method.* Philadelphia, Westminster Press, 1982.
15. Chambers, Oswald. *My Utmost for His Highest.* New York, Dodd, Mead, 1935.
16. Weil, Simone. *Waiting on God.* Glasgow, William Collins Sons, 1951.
17. Baxter, Richard. *Poetical Fragments*. Quoted in Pooley, Roger and Seddon, Philip (Eds.), *The Lord of the Journey,* London, Collins, 1986.
18. Donne, John. "Sermon preached at Pauls upon Christmas Day in the evening, 1624," *The Sermons of John Donne*, Vol. VI, Potter, George R. & Simpson, Evelyn M. (Eds.), Berkeley, University of California Press, 1953.

Osler's Gamble and Ours:
The Meaning of Contempory History*

Daniel Michael Fox

Since 1990 **Daniel M. Fox** has been President of the Milbank Memorial Fund, the nation's oldest endowed foundation in health care and public health. Prior to that he was a faculty member and administrator at Harvard University, and then at the Health Sciences Center of the State University of New York at Stony Brook. He has served in state government in Massachusetts and New York, and as an advisor to or staff member of several federal agencies. Fox holds A.B., A.M. and Ph.D. degrees from Harvard University, and is a member of the Institute of Medicine of the National Academy of Sciences and of the Council on Foreign Relations.

In addition to articles in journals of health affairs, social science and history, Dr. Fox has written *Power and Illness: The Failure and Future of American Health Policy* (1993 and 1995); *Engines of Culture* (1963 and 1994)*; The Discovery of Abundance* (1967 and 2002); *Economists and Health Care* (1979); *Health Politics, Health Policies: The Experience of Britain and America 1911-1965* (1986); and *Photographing Medicine: Images and Power in Britain and America since 1840* (1988). He co-edited *AIDS: The Burdens of His tory* (1988); *AIDS: The Making of a Chronic Disease* (1992); *Five States That Could Not Wait: Lessons for Health Reform from Florida, Hawaii, Minnesota, Oregon and Vermont* (1994); *Home-Based Care for a New Century* (1996); and *Treating Drug Abusers Effectively* (1996).

*Delivered 10 April 1991 at the Twenty-first Annual Meeting of the American Osler Society, New Orleans, Louisiana

"Osler's Gamble"? Some members of the American Osler Society may be surprised at the title of this paper. How could a man who believed so strongly in the methods of science be a gambler? The answer is that what Osler did as a result of his belief in the power of science was a gamble, though many historians and admirers of Osler might prefer to call it an investment. (Some of them may also think that buying stock or awarding academic tenure is an investment.) Osler bet that the contemporary history of medicine, events that occurred during the last half of the nineteenth century, taught lessons about the future. He very deliberately used an interpretation of events in the recent past as the basis for advocating how his contemporaries ought to organize the practice of medicine, medical education, and research. Osler, that is, demonstrated the practical value of studying the history of medicine.

The purpose of this paper is to address two questions that follow from this assertion. The first question is: What use did Osler make of the contemporary history of medicine? The second question is more controversial: What does Osler's use of his contemporary history suggest about how we should use our own?

Osler studied the history of medicine in the nineteenth century, and used it as the basis for his predictions about medicine in the twentieth century. Then he worked hard to make what he had predicted happen. History became a basic science, in a sense, of his advocacy.

Contrast this to how most physicians, even distinguished physicians, approach the history of medicine in the late twentieth century. They do not study it. Their predictions about medicine in the twenty-first century, when they make them, are based on beliefs about recent events that are rarely based on systematic research and analysis. History, far from being a basic science of advocacy, is hardly noticed by most of the people I have met in the two decades during which I have been from time to time a medical school faculty member, a manager in an academic health center, a public official, and a foundation executive.

Thus my story has a moral. Osler gambled that medicine in the twentieth century would be shaped by the lessons he chose to draw from the history of medicine in the nineteenth century. If we want to gamble on the shape of medicine in the twenty-first century, we could improve our odds by drawing lessons from the history of medicine in the twentieth century.

This story has two parts. One is about Osler. The other is about us. Osler once neatly summed up the purpose of both parts: "It is one of the values of lectures on the history of medicine to keep alive the good influences of great men even after their positive teaching is antiquated."[1]

Osler's Gamble

Osler was quite precise about what he believed to be the most important theme in the history of medicine. Several times and famously in 1913, he said that this theme was the "progressive evolution of scientific medicine."[2] He believed that the history of medicine before his own time was characterized by a lengthy "series of upward steps." These steps, he also called them "stages," were as follows. First, medicine "emerged from magic and religion into an empirical art." Then the "natural character of disease was recognized and the importance of its study as a phenomenon of nature was announced." Next the "structure and functions of the human body were worked out." After that, the "clinical and anatomical features of disease were determined." Then the "causes of disorders were profitably studied." In sum, "science has completely changed man's attitude toward disease."[3]

He had earlier been quite precise about what he meant by science and about how science had changed attitudes toward disease. A convenient summary of his views was his talk in 1901 on "Medicine in the Nineteenth Century." The nineteenth century was, he said, "wonderful" because the "phenomenal results which have followed *experimental investigations*," promised " . . . the decrease of physical suffering in man, woman and child when stricken by disease or accident." He then described, disease by disease, recent advances in medical knowledge and their practical consequences.[4]

In 1901, Osler asserted that the most important result of the recent history of science, especially of physiology and pathology, was "to emancipate medicine from routine and the thraldom of authority."[5] At the end of his life he extended the reach of this generalization to include the study of history. "History," he wrote in 1917, "teaches us the growth and development of ideas." Two sets of ideas, two "master thoughts of the race," were centrally important to understanding history and its practical consequences. The first set of ideas was the history of religious thought. The other was ideas about "knowledge of things we see, patiently acquired by searching out the secrets of nature." This knowledge was the "basis of our material civilization." In particular the "new biology" had, in his lifetime, changed the "mental outlook" of thoughtful members of the human race.[6]

I have summarized this familiar Osleriana in order to emphasize four points that are central to my thesis about the relevance of Osler's gamble to the gambles that we could make. The first point is the vast importance that Osler accorded to history as basic to an understanding of medicine. The second point is his commitment to a clearly articulated and systematic interpretation of the history of medicine. Not for Osler a view of history as whatever facts and anecdotes somebody remembers. Third, he was convinced that history was driven by ideas. Fourth, ideas, especially scientific ideas, could liberate medicine, and by extension other areas of life, from two tyrannies that Osler loathed—the tyranny of routine and the tyranny of authority

Osler used these four points as the basis for his gamble. That is, he extracted from them an analysis of current events. Then he used this analysis to guide, prospectively, his behavior as a physician. In the language of my clinical profession of public administration, Osler used history as the basis for policy. By policy, I mean both his behavior as a clinician and as a professor and his advice to the people who managed and subsidized medical education.

I call Osler's use of history for policy a gamble because it was prospective. Osler acted on what he took to be the lessons of history in what we now call real time. Osler described his gamble quite precisely. The task of subsequent historians is to evaluate it.

There are many primary sources for documenting Osler's gamble. I choose two of them to make my case. In one the gamble is implicit, in the other explicit.

The gamble is implicit in the second part of "The Fixed Period." This essay has been interpreted by scholars who know considerably more about Osler than I do. I simply want to suggest that, among his other goals in this essay, Osler was doing something that most policy makers do: he was trying to influence how his contemporaries and their successors would evaluate his gamble. Thus he describes the importance of the Johns Hopkins Hospital and medical school for contemporary history. He urges his listeners and subsequent readers to agree that, in its short history, these institutions had linked four important goals. The first goal was to emphasize the "importance of scientific investigation of disease." The second was to make explicit that the hospital was a place for the "study as well as for the cure of disease." The third, which followed from the first two, was to demonstrate that a teaching hospital required a "vital organic connection with a university." And the fourth was to exemplify, the "advantages of well trained doctors to a community."[7]

In order to make Osler's gamble clear to you, I will translate these four goals into the language of late twentieth century health policy. In our language, Osler's goals sound something like this: Any rational health policy for any country gives priority to academic medicine. It does so because improvements in the health status of any population or individual will be produced a) by laboratory research, b) by a teaching hospital that can provide both the material for laboratory research and the patients on which to test what is learned in laboratories, and c) by doctors practicing in community settings who have learned about diagnosis, treatment and prevention in teaching hospitals that are linked to modern scientific universities.

Now let us return to the early twentieth century, and therefore to the language of Osler and his contemporaries. About a year after he wrote "The Fixed Period," Osler was explicit about his policy gamble in the introduction to a multivolume text he edited with Thomas McRae, *A System of Medicine: Its Theory and Practice*. Like any accomplished policy gambler, moreover, Osler used shrewd tactics to persuade his audience to accept his logic.

Osler begins his introduction by reciting his fundamental lessons of history. First, he insists that history changes as the result of ideas. This theme, that ideas are the motor of history, is, we know from other texts, Osler's code for asserting the virtues of analytical thinking against the tacky claims of routine and authority. He then reminds his readers that "scientific medicine," which began among the Greeks in the fifth and sixth centuries was the "product of a union of religion with philosophy." Now he moves to the scientific triumphs of the late nineteenth century. He describes how the new ability to detect the specific etiology of infectious diseases led to advances in "sanitary control," and in "vaccines, antitoxins and curative sera."[8]

Sanitary control? Osler seems to be placing at least a side bet on public health, or maybe he was making a different policy gamble than the one that was so close to the surface of "The Fixed Period." But look more closely at his tactics of argument. He now says that "in the immediate future it is along chemical lines that we may look for the greatest advance . . ." in useful scientific knowledge.[9] He has embraced readers who believe that public health policy matters, but he has pushed them toward agreeing that sanitary control is driven by laboratory science.

He continues the same tactics on the next page. Again he seems to be hedging his bet when he says that ". . . upon diet more than upon any other single factor depends the health of the community."[10] He seems to be saying that good health policy includes social policy to improve nutrition.

But wait: A masterful gambler is working to make other people place the same bets that he has made. A few lines later, he flatters the people who do the "daily work in general practice," calling them the "hope of the profession."[11]

Suddenly he shifts the argument. He is ready to make his policy gamble explicit. Osler's transition to a full statement of his gamble requires him to make plain that he is a *physician scientist*. He and his allies will fail if they do not mould the general practitioners whom he has just flattered in their own image. Thus "our labors are in vain—all the manifold contributions of science . . . unless the result in making men better able to fight the battle against disease."[12]

Now Osler is ready to state his policy gamble without qualification. "Gradually," he says, "almost insensibly, the practical advances of the *laboratory* and of the *hospital* reach the men with whom . . . rests the final testing of our efforts." Even public health and nutrition are within the scope of practice of general practitioners, not of public health policy. Thus the "work in practical sanitation, the last word in the prevention of disease" as well as the "carrying out of new methods of treatment" rest with the "rank and file of the profession."[13]

Making explicit the basis of his gamble on the meanings—the significance for policy—of contemporary history, Osler next says that because the "times are changing" policy must change. He explicitly calls this policy "a reorganization" of power and influence in internal medicine and declares that its basis must be the dominance of highly trained internists in teaching hospitals that are linked both to laboratory researchers and to community practitioners. Then he ends his argument by changing the tense of his appeal to historical analysis: the "times [he says] have changed."[14]

Our Gamble

Times have indeed changed yet again. Therefore I invite the members of the American Osler Society, and other colleagues, to address two questions, one retrospective, the other prospective. The historical question is this: How successful was Osler as a gambler? The prospective question is what principal bets, and what side bets would you like to place on health policy for the early twenty-first century? I will amplify these questions, and then encourage you to discuss them with me and then with each other.

First, how successful was Osler's gamble? It is obvious that Osler and his allies were persuasive. There is a rich literature, some of it the work of members of this Society that describes how scientific physicians came to dominate medicine in the United States in the twentieth century. We know the familiar history of medical schools and teaching hospitals, of the specialties and the subspecialties, and of the financing and structure of medical research. We have also heard the complaints, throughout the century, of many of the people who were relegated to secondary importance in the hierarchies of power and the hierarchies of values on which Osler and his allies placed their bets. I refer, for example, to several well-documented conflicts between town and gown, between generalists and specialists, between Oslerean gamblers and advocates of according high priority to primary care in medical education and health care financing, and between specialists on public health and almost everybody of influence in medicine.

How you will answer my first question, how successful Osler's gamble was, depends on how you evaluate these conflicts among competing claimants to power and authority in medicine. Would the health status of the American people in 1991 have been different if the Oslerean gamble had not paid off so well in funds for basic research, in the proliferation of teaching hospital beds and services, and in specialization? Would the health status of Americans be any different if the people who wanted to place different bets between 1890 and 1920 had been more successful in influencing the allocation of power and of moral authority in medicine and in health policy?

Evaluating the success of Osler's gamble also means evaluating his historiography. That is, might Osler have placed a different bet if he had read history differently. You will recall that, in Osler's historiography, ideas drive the events of history. To him, the central ideas in history are religion and science. In the nineteenth century the idea of science generated advances that promised to lead to vast improvements in the health of populations.

But what if different ideas drove history? Consider, for example, what we have learned since the nineteenth century about the power of the idea of tribal loyalty in its modern form of nationalism or about the power of religious belief and ideology to put to dreadful uses the ideas of science and their translation into, for example, war-making technology.

And what if history is not driven mainly by ideas at all?

What if it is driven by the conflicts of classes that are formed in response to the social relations of production? What if history is driven by greed, or fear, or hatred as well as by ideas? If history is, pardon the expression, multi-factorial, how would we have placed better bets than Osler's in order to reduce mortality and morbidity in our country, or in anybody else's?

I will be specific about the relevance of these questions to the history of medicine, and particularly to the history of the broad issues I am calling health policy. Osler's gamble was based on his conviction that a particular set of ideas that drove history in the past should be the principal determinant of health policy in the future. Thus he chose not to worry about how two other large matters would influence the results of his gamble. One of these matters was *interests*. One example of interests is how members of the medical profession have acted on what they took to be their economic and psychological needs during this century. Another example of interests is what employers and the elected representatives of the people have believed it is important to pay for in order to maintain and improve health.

Illness is, surprisingly, another large matter that Osler left out of his historiography and therefore out of the calculations that led to his gamble. Osler's gamble did not take account of potential changes in the epidemiological situation: changes driven by the advances of science, and by changes in the economy, in demography and in living patterns. Shortly after Osler's death, chronic diseases became, for the first time in recorded statistics, the leading causes of death among Americans.[15] By the 1990s, managing disability attendant to aging, injury, and chronic disease had become, to many people, a more pressing problem for health policy than prolonging life or reducing pain. How would Osler have gambled if he had imagined that such a vast change would occur in the epidemiological and demographic situation over the next several generations?

Which, of course, leads me to ask my second question: What bets will you place, using what historical analysis that is grounded in what historiography? Osler gambled intelligently, that is, he was explicit about the analytical basis of his bet. Not for Osler a random walk either down Wall Street or into the future. Will we be so intelligent?

We have no choice about whether we will gamble. We place bets on health policy every time we take a political action, whether that action is in the relatively closed politics of professional practice or in the relatively open politics of health care financing and organization. The question is how to bet, not whether to bet.

Neither do we have any choice about whether we will use history in placing our bets on the future.[16] The only question is whether we will be more or less sophisticated than Osler in using it. Perhaps we cannot even aspire to Osler's level of historical sophistication.

The alternative to using history in our policy gambles, is to assume naively that what is happening around us today is likely to continue to happen. This is the famous view that history is just one damn thing after another. Such a view would be inconsistent with being in this room, although I suspect that each of us has colleagues who routinely act on it.

I hope that I have said enough to stimulate discussion. I would like to hear your views about both Osler's gamble and the gambles that we may make. Here is what I propose as a method of procedure. I will moderate a discussion that will, I hope, be so lively that I have to cut it off after twenty minutes. During the discussion I will make as few comments as possible—and those will be intended mainly to increase clarity in discussion. Then I will pause for a minute or two to collect my thoughts about what you have been saying about the uses of contemporary history and the sorts of gambles you are prepared to make. That is, I will behave like the contemporary historian that I am and use our discussion as my primary source material.

> [A vigorous discussion occurred among the members of the American Osler Society. During the discussion the author deliberately turned his back on the audience and took public notes on a large pad that he had placed on an easel below the lectern. The notes were in red marker. After twenty minutes, the author analyzed the notes, using a black marker to circle key words and concepts. Then he returned to the lectern to complete his presentation.]

Like Osler, most of the members of the American Osler Society in 1991 are eager to use history prospectively to gamble. But they read primary sources differently than Osler did and, therefore, reach conclusions that are more pessimistic than his. They draw three generalizations about the future from recent history. The first is that, contrary to what Osler and many of his contemporaries believed, progress in medicine is neither inevitable nor linear.

The second generalization is that the context of medicine has changed. Osler gambled that physicians, and especially physician-scientists, could shape medical practice by the force of their ideas and their ability to control the dominant institutions of the profession. There are now more actors and interests. Events in economic and social life, in the environment and even in foreign affairs are shaping the future of medicine. As one person said, "social chips" are now part of the gamble; Osler could play only "scientific chips." Moreover, the relationship between science and technology, which Osler believed to be straightforward, is now seen as complicated, especially as a result of the mediating force of industrial interests. The future of technology and its influence on medicine often seems to be unpredictable.

The third generalization is that money matters in medicine, now and in the future, much more than it did for Osler. Of course physicians in the past, and Osler himself, took money seriously and enjoyed immensely earning a lot of it. But payment, more precisely the policies of payers, will increasingly determine physicians' behavior in the future in ways that were unthinkable in the past.

Finally, several members of the group voiced profound doubts about whether the future of medicine could be gambled on at all. One spoke of the "irrationality of man." Another wondered if "any historical system has meaning."

Bets having been placed and recorded, I stepped down from the lectern. Perhaps at some future date the gamblers will revisit the casino of prospective history.[17]

References

1. Osler, W. *The Evoloution of Modern Medicine.* A series of Lectures Delivered at Yale University on the Silliman Foundation in April, 1913. New Haven, CT, Yale University Press, 1921, p. 219.
2. Ibid., p. 223.
3. Ibid., pp. 220-221.
4. Osler, W. "Medicine in the Nineteenth Century," in *Aequanimitas With Other Addresses to Medical Students, Nurses, and Practitioners of Medicine,* Philadelphia, P. Blakiston's Son, 3rd ed., 1932, pp. 219-224.
5. Ibid., p. 223.
6. Osler, W. "Introduction" to Charles Singer (Ed.), *Studies in the History, and Method of Science,* Oxford, Clarendon Press, 1917.
7. Osler, W. "The Fixed Period," reprinted in *Aequanimitas*. Originally published as "Valedictory Address at Johns Hopkins University, " JAMA 44: 705-710, 1905.
8. Osler, W. and McRae, T. (Eds.). *A System of Medicine, Its Theory and Practice.* Vol. I London, Williams and Norgate, 1907, pp. xvii-xviii.
9. Ibid., p. xviii.
10. Ibid., p. xxix.
11. Ibid., p. xxix.
12. Ibid., p. xxix.
13. Ibid., p. xxix.
14. Ibid., pp. xxxiii-xxxiv.
15. Fox, D.M. "Health Policy and Changing Epidemiology in the United States: Chronic Disease in the Twentieth Century," in Maulitz, R. (Ed.). *Unnatural Causes, The Three Leading Killer Diseases in America*. New Brunswick, Rutgers University Press, 1989; Fox, D.M. "Policy and Epidemiology Financing Health Services for the Chronically Ill and Disabled, 1930-1990."

The Milbank Quarterly, 67: Supplement 2, part 2: 257-287, 1989

16. The metaphor of a random walk comes from a modern classic about gambles on history, Malkiel, B.C. *A Random Walk Down Wall Street.* 5th ed., New York, W.W. Norton, 1991.

The author thanks Drs. Richard L. Golden and Kenneth M. Ludmerer for assistance in locating primary sources generated by Osler.

From Doctor to Nurse with Love in a Molecular Age*

William C. Beck

William C. Beck was Born in Chicago, Illinois, in 1907, and educated at the University of Wisconsin and Northwestern University (B.A., M.D.). Following residency training in Frankfurt, a/m Germany, he practiced as a general surgeon in Chicago,. He was on the staff of the St. Joseph and St. Vincent Hospitals in Chicago, as well as the Cook County and Illinois Research Hospitals. He taught at the University of Illinois until entrance into the U.S. Army with the Cook County Hospital Affiliated 297th General Hospital in World War II. He also served as Chief of the Surgical Services with the Syracuse University Unit and at Gardiner General Hospital with the rank of Colonel. Following the war, Dr. Beck joined the Guthrie Clinic in Sayre, Pennsylvania, eventually becoming Chief of the Department of Surgery of the Robert Packer Hospital and Guthrie Clinic. He was a lecturer in Surgery at the University of Pennsylvania and Professor of Surgery at Hahnemann University. He died in 1994.

Dr. Beck's research interests were in the area of surgical infection control, and the other elements in the surroundings of the hospital such as lighting, air currents, air conditioning, and the delivery of health care. His books include *Health Care Environment* (1982), and *Memory Bytes: An Autobiography of a Surgeon* (1995). He also published numerous articles and reviews.

Dr. Beck was President Emeritus of the Guthrie Foundation for Education and Research, President of the Association for the Advancement of Medical Instrumentation, Chairman of the Health Fa cilities Committee of the Illuminating Engineering Society of North America, and a member of committees of the American Standards

*Delivered 26 March 1992 at the Twenty-second Annual Meeting of the American Osler Society, San Diego, California.

Institute, American Society for Testing and Materials, and American College of Surgeons. Dr. Beck also was a member of the American Surgical Association, Societe International de Chirugie, Central Society for Clinical Research, Central Surgical Association, Chicago Surgical Society, Royal Society of Medicine (England), and the American Medical Association.

I am indeed most honored to be asked to make a presentation to your prestigious group. Unfortunately my medical education did not include the best and best known work in medicine, the Osler Principles. But, for many years, at least weekly I do consult the *Bibliotheca Osleriana*. These thumbed pages, are within easy reach from my desk. It is, as you all know, not a pure reference volume, but contains a most thoughtful commentary. Thus it always provides stimulus, and inspiration to even the most modest lover of books. I have, recently, reread parts of *Aequanimitas*. The beauty of his writing I had forgotten, and I am grateful for this stimulus to renew my reading.

The pride I feel at presenting a lecture in the name of Dr. John P. McGovern is an expression of the many wonderful tributes published in 1980 by the Health Sciences Institute.

Dr. McGovern with Dr. Henderson, in describing the origin of your Society, said that one of its aims is to counter what Sir William described as "Medical Chauvinism." It is to this end that I have chosen to review the past, present and possible future interrelationships between the two principal healing professions, medicine and nursing.

The practice of medicine as espoused by Sir William Osler no longer exists. It is not even the sole domain of the medical doctor. The practice of allergy as the vocation of Dr. McGovern is no longer the exclusive realm of the physician allergist. Medical practice has evolved into a host of subdisciplines. For example, allergy is now the joint endeavor of allergists, immunologists, molecular biologists, aeropollution counters, medical technologists, and office nurses; although the allergist's name may still be the only one on the office door.

This metamorphosis has taken place during my own life span. When I left medical school, the famous painting by Sir Luke Fildes entitled "The Doctor" typified our profession.[1] The bearded physician sits sympathetically beside a sick child lying on two mismatched chairs. The parents anxiously watch in the dimly lighted room, while the doctor obviously wonders what to do. Today's scientist M.D., Ph.D., (probably also bearded) in a well-illuminated hospital setting, has reviewed a host of imaging and laboratory reports and consulted computerized algorithms. He is confident and knows exactly what to do. He has at hand a library with access to the world literature, consultants for every detail, and a compendium of unpronounceable miracle drugs.

Specialization, of course, is *per se* not modern. Lyons and Petrucelli[2] report that Heroditus, in the fifth century B.C. wrote this of Egyptian medicine,

> Medicine with them is distributed in the following way: every physician is for one disease and not for several, and the whole country is of physicians of the eyes; others for the head; others for the teeth; others for the belly and others of obscure diseases.

They go on to say that specialization was not necessarily evidence of an advanced system of medicine, but that the Hermetic Collection of writings was so great that to learn it all would have been too great for any one man. Of course, this is, in large part, the reason for our fragmentation of practice today. It is my belief, and the subject of this dissertation that, while we have witnessed an explosion of this specialization process, economics will drive us into a countervailing implosion. The shrinking of multifactorial medicine will, I believe, be driven by the cost of superspecialization and by a shift of responsibility. The latter is attained by the transfer of tasks from doctor to nurse. As we shall see, this has already been and is continuing to be taking place.

The development of these phenomena can be traced through history. Medical practice progressed sluggishly until the middle of the eighteenth century. The medicine described by Galen in the second century had been practiced until 1700. Dr. Osler said: "Galen so read the meaning of Hippocrates that for fifteen centuries medicine stopped thinking." Artists Leonardo da Vinci and Albrecht Dürer led the way into the new medicine. The turning point came with Semmelweis and Nightingale. In the middle of the eighteenth century, Ignaz Semmelweis evolved the method which made a hospital a safe place in which to give birth. He developed the simple precept of having attendants bathe their hands in a chlorine antiseptic rather than ineffectually washing them in a dirty basin.[3] This reduced the hospital mortality from about 12 percent to 1 percent. During the same decade, Miss Florence Nightingale made hospitals safe for war casualties by introducing sanitation, ventilation, and nutrition. This reduced the mortality in Skutari from 42 percent to 2 percent.[4] These feats are probably the only ones which would fit Lloyd MacLean of McGill's "Lead Ball Principle." He is quoted as saying, "If you hold a lead ball out the window and when you let go it goes up, you don't need a statistician to tell you that it was a significant event."[5] The same decade also saw the beginnings of anesthesia, and identified the relationship between bacteria to infection.

A new era came into being following the Semmelweis and Nightingale innovations. All science seems to have acquired a new impetus. The benefits of publication seemingly were fully employed, achieving a global circulation of new ideas. The next landmark was World War II. Then an outburst of science took place and it is still in progress. Our learning is expanding logarithmically. I believe that much of this is due to miniaturization and new methods to display images. The light microscope provided knowledge of the cell and its diseases. The electron microscope revealed the anatomy and physiology of the cell itself. At present "researchers can measure and manipulate subcellular elements too small to be seen by the most powerful magnification."[6]

We have now entered into a molecular age. Cellular and molecular manipulation has today become a part of clinical medicine and is flourishing in the laboratory as well. Technology has even progressed to the point where it is possible to recognize individual elements employing X-ray microanalysis. Here individual atoms are struck by electrons which results in the emission of X-rays. These are diffracted into types recognizable for every element. For study with the scanning electron microscope, tissues or even non-biologic material can be replicated into sections only a few tenths of a nanometer thick. Only a very few years ago our sections were cut with a microtome. I even learned to cut sections by hand, and you might imagine their thickness.

Medical education has kept pace with this current practice. Years have been added to the development of the physician. Medical school curricula have become standardized. Acceptance of the advances of basic science research alters teaching as it largely is produced by the same educators. Years of additional schooling and practical application through residency are demanded before permitting independent 'practice' on patients.

Even with the added years required there is almost a full supply of physicians. Some even say that there is an oversupply. In contrast, there has always been a huge need for nurses. In 1948, an A.M.A. committee reported that nursing schools needed to double their enrollment to provide a minimum supply. In that report 63 percent of hospitals were in very short supply.[7] This situation has continued to the present time. The current need is exemplified by the tremendous inducements offered in the classified sections of our media. As a result, more and more nurse substitutes have come into being: nursing assistants, technicians in all fields, etc. This undersupply has caused those organizations and institutions who needed nurses most to discourage the educational progress which medicine has enjoyed.

Nursing history is as old as that of medicine. Lyons and Petrucelli[8] quote Charaka's Samhita who, in India, a millennium before Christ, listed four qualifications for a nurse: "knowledge of the manner in which medicines should be prepared or compounded; cleverness; devotion to the patient; and purity of mind and body." Osler lists "...the mystic seven, your lamps to lighten, tact, tidiness, taciturnity, sympathy, gentleness, cheerfulness all linked together by charity."

They go on to state that, during the crusades, orders of friars performed nursing duties. This would dispel the notion that nursing historically had always been limited to females.

Miss Nightingale's contribution included the creation of schooled professionals (unfortunately dubbed 'trained' rather than 'educated.'). No longer would nursing service be provided by domestic servants.[9] Nuns, who had taken over the duties of the friars now also instituted 'training.'

Since nursing's first claim to professional status, they have been gradually achieving its true dimension. This has been accomplished through necessity rather than protest. World economics has required the creation of a *new* nurse; one to whom increasing professional responsibility can be entrusted. They have proven themselves fully worthy. Moreover, it has engendered the respect that they seek. William Knaus and colleagues, have shown that the cooperative effort of physician and nurse is reflected in reduction of morbidity, mortality, and patient suffering.[10]

However, the Knaus study also revealed that the successful nurse contributor to the partnership is a *very well educated* (not trained) one. "Clinical specialists with *master's degrees* and extensive experience in intensive care had as their primary responsibility the orientation and development of the nursing staff."

Quite in contrast, the basic R.N. status can today be achieved by any one of three routes, lasting either two, three or four years. The four-year course leads to a Bachelor of Nursing degree; the R.N. comes through a credentialing examination. I have, in 1964, suggested that nursing must reorient their educational system. I said that only one standard should exist.[11]

Although nursing's educational standards may not have kept pace, the incursion of certifiable specialization has, in the last few years, transformed nursing practice. Unfortunately, the Nursing Specialty Boards do not inspect and accredit the institutions which provide the post-R.N. training.[12] The specialties to which nurses may be accredited are growing as rapidly as are the Medical Boards. It might be well to recall Dr. Charles H. Mayo's aphorism that "the definition of a specialist is one who knows more about less and less." Not as well known is his added caveat "it is essential that the specialist must have some association with others who represent the whole of which the specialty is a part."[13] I would add that the nurse educator should be a person of superior education (which Knaus defines as a person with an advanced collegiate degree[10]). Most Nursing Boards state (1993) they will accept only R.N.s who have at least a baccalaureate degree.[12]

I must now address the very difficult question of interprofessional dissonance. That it is significant is attested by the fact that a search of the national literature discloses that ninty-three articles in both nursing and medical refereed literature addressed this issue during the last year. Most suggest that nurses have been forced to truckle to the physician; surgeons demand a fawning, obsequious *female* yielding to their apotheotic demands. Some have suggested that the relationship has become a "game."[14] Others feel that a special partnership should exist between nurse and patient,[15] [not the physician]. That the nurse is the patient's 'advocate', and should 'blow the whistle' on incompetent physicians.[16] I found *none* that recognized that the patient could discharge his doctor, but could not fire his nurse. Also that an 'advocate' is customarily chosen by the person represented, unless assigned by a court; even then the client has a choice.

I, however, do believe that the nurse/doctor contentions will gradually disappear as the hospital-based nurse becomes a more important *partner* in the care team. Today's young physician has survived a course of four years of premedical study and four years of medical school, then an internship. During his next four or five years of residency, he may appear condescending or even overbearing to the nurse. But as he mellows and recognizes the accomplishments of the nursing teammate, arrogance will be replaced by appreciation.

The Nurse Practice Act in my Commonwealth of Pennsylvania[17] defines nursing as follows: "The practice of professional nursing means diagnosing and treating human responses to actual or potential health problems through such services as case finding, health teaching, health counseling, and provision of care supportive to or restorative of life and well being *and executing medical regimens as prescribed by a licensed physician or dentist"* [italics are mine]. The latter portion of the definition is a point of contact between professional nurse and physician in which dissonance might occur, because the physician does not recognize, nor possibly appreciate the many other services rendered by the modern professional nurse.

From time to time, the State Board of Nursing proposes rules and regulations, ratified by the State Legislature, which are descriptive of the changing aspects of some of the clinical nursing activities. So, for example, our State Legal Code cites the following examples: "To collect arterial and venous blood even in adult and infant intensive care units; carry out vaginal examinations and do 'Pap' smears; do certain intraocular procedures; remove sutures; practice hypnosis; program pacemakers; use and administer drugs, administer chemotherapy; and change tracheostomy and gastrostomy tubes."[18] In California, they may now write prescriptions. These, not too long ago, were considered solely the province of an advanced chief resident in his fourth or fifth year. My own chief, my father, and Dr. Osler as well as others of that generation are spinning in their graves. But the modern Professional nurse has proven to be fully equal to these tasks, and carries them out deftly and with aplomb.

When I recently entered a hospital as a patient, a nurse recorded my history and physically examined me. She sent an aide to take my temperature, count respiration, and take my blood pressure. She also instructed a student nurse in how to insert a venous catheter and start an intravenous solution. My surgeon examined the anatomy of his proposed operation and read the nurse's chart. The junior resident recorded the therapeutic plan for my illness. She did find time to explain what was in store for me.

The surgeon turned over to the nurse my clinical management both before and after the operation. She (or he) bestowed on me most of the 'tender loving care' that I received. A nursing assistant carried on most of what Miss Nightingale had defined as "nursing." A dietitian discussed with me my diabetic diet, the respiratory technician my breathing, a radiology technician took my X-ray, ultrasound, and magnetic resonance scans. In these days of molecular science, the physician serves the functions of 'Mission Control' at Cape Canaveral, while the nurse acts as the astronaut. A host of well-trained technicians and technologists make this possible. As an 'outpatient' I had a prolonged course of radiation therapy. A Therapeutic Radiologist designed the treatment plan, and a physicist calculated the proper alignments to produce the required dosage with a minimum of skin exposure. The daily adjustment of the huge linear accelerator and the placement of my anatomy into the proper alignment was done by technicians who turned the gadget on and off.

My illness provided me with a 'catbird seat' to observe the current hospital practice. It appears that health care is becoming ever more hierarchal. In my early days, *all* of the clinical care was carried out by the physician. Nurses performed the non-clinical functions as well as the housekeeping. The education emerging from Miss Nightingale's contributions,[19] as well as the realization of the nurse's capabilities has redefined the functional parameters. Without doubt, these will continue to change.

What would Dr. Osler have thought of the current system? According to Richard Golden, in his presidential address two years ago, Dr. Osler was characterized as a therapeutic nihilist. I believe he belonged to the second generation of modern medicine based on pathology; the first rested on anatomy. The third, from which we are presently emerging, is concerned with normal and abnormal physiology. Dr. Osler would probably decry our present concentration on therapy. But today we have specific treatment for almost all bacterial disease. Our present concern is with certain viruses.

Sir William's opinions of nursing seem less clear. Of Florence Nightingale he said "Ever blessed be her name." Of nursing in general he wrote "A luxury in private, the trained nurse has become one of the blessings of humanity, taking a place between physician and priest: And not inferior to either." But he also said "Darwin gives a graphic account of the marvelous care-taking capacity of the little *Formica fusca*—a slave ant."

Today's most vexing and significant problem is to expand the supply of nurses, and to enrich and standardize their education. These imperatives must be accomplished simultaneously. Now education and supply vie for priority, each at the expense of the other. Hospitals, those who need nurses, seek a reduction in the requirements for the R.N. Nursing organizations attempt to augment education at the sacrifice of supply. Educational advancement and other techniques are being offered to lure more into the nursing profession, as well as to entice nurses to their own institution as you can see in the classified pages of our print media.[20] This at a time when there is massive unemployment, including females, with literally millions seeking jobs.

I might suggest a possible solution. It would involve a restructuring of the entire entry system into the nursing pyramid. It would be accomplished by giving academic credit for each of the progressive stages of development. So, for example, a young lady could enter the health care field at any level. She might begin with the educational curriculum for nurses' aids. After graduation and serving in this endeavor for a minimum time, she could apply to a course for nurses' assistants or technicians, getting credit to an advanced standing in that curriculum. After service at that level, she could apply for advanced standing in a school of 'practical' nursing. Graduation from one of these might qualify for advanced standing in an academic school of nursing. After graduation from nursing school, armed with prescribed activity in an "accredited" training program, she could qualify for a specialty certification examination. Thus, each of the ladder's steps would recognize previous attainments. Each of these schools would have to have a minimum curriculum approved by the State's Nursing Board.

Such a system would legitimize the nursing hierarchy, establish goals to be set by each individual. Entry could be at any level, and progress from one to the other could be monitored. I believe that it would attract many more into the field as they view their potentials. I have used the gender consideration, because nursing's parameters are ones in which women have been able to not only excel, but their attainments have been recognized. Also 97 percent of nurses are women. Furthermore, we are seeing a tremendous increase in the number of women achieving positions of excellence and reward in all of health care.

This concept is essentially not original. Alt and Housten have written a book on the subject.[21] The University of Texas M.D. Anderson Hospital has created career ladders in their own instructional systems. It divides all levels of nursing into five steps, with definitions for each, and progress from one into another. In our area, a Community College has a cooperative arrangement with a State University where an associate degree can be extended to a Bachelor of Science from one to the other. What I believe is new is suggesting this method for general adoption and specifically as a recruitment tool to significantly add to the nursing pool as an objective.

I agree with George Weinstein who characterized the ideal professional as one "who is compassionate, skillful, knowledgeable and creative."[22] This applies to both physician and nurse. Nurses are now greeting patients and introducing themselves by name. Unfortunately, this is often as Alice or Jane, rather than Alice Jones or Jane Smith. One has to dislocate one's neck to read the name tag through the lower segment of one's trifocals. But nurses are responsibly accepting the challenges and obligations of clinical care gracefully and efficiently. I believe that more and more complex duties will come under their purview, and will be well handled. As this proceeds, the relationships will develop into mutual trust and respect. This process will be beneficial to the patient, who is already a mutual responsibility. The professions will, in my judgment, intertwine as do the snakes on the caduceus. This, I hope, will continue to develop as we progress into the molecular age.[23]

References

1. The original hangs in the lobby of the Robert Packer Hospital in Sayre, PA. A second version in the Tate Gallery in London. The two paintings were exhibited together at the Manchester City Art Gallery in November - January 1987-1988.
2. Lyons, A.S. and Petrucelli, R.J. *Medicine: An Illustrated History.* New York, Abradale Press, Harry N. Abrams, 1987, p. 101.
3. Beck, W.C. Handwashing, Semmelweis, and Chlorine. *Infect Control Hosp Epidemiol* 9: 366-367, 1988.
4. Bettmann. O.L. *A Pictorial History of Medicine.* Springfield, IL, Charles C. Thomas, 1956, p. 268.
5. Del Guercio, L.R.M. Septic Shock, Monoclonal Antibodies, and the Lead Ball Principle. *Complications in Surg* 10: 10, 1991.
6. Swerdlow, J.L. A New Kind of Kinship. *National Geographic.* 180: 64-92, 1991.
7. Organization Section, Ad Hoc Committee on Nursing Report. *JAMA*, 137: 878-879, 1948.
8. Op. cit. #1, p. 112.
9. Nightingale, F. *Notes on Nursing: What it is and What it is Not*. Philadelphia, Lippincott, 1957 [London, Original Harrison & Sons 1859].
10. Knaus, W.A., Draper, E.A., Wagner, D.P. An evaluation of outcome from intensive care in major medical centers. *Ann Int Med* 104: 410-415, 1986.
11. Beck, W.C. Medicine and Nursing. *Surg Gynec & Obstet* 119: 593, 1964.
12. American Nurses Credentialing Center: Professional Certification. *Certification Catalog.* American Nurses Association, 2420 Pershing Road, Kansas City, MO. 64108.
13. Willius, F.A., Mayo, C.H. and Mayo, W.J. *Aphorisms of Dr. Charles Horace Mayo, 1865-1939 and Dr. William James Mayo, 1861-1939.* Springfield, IL, Charles C. Thomas, 1951.
14. Stein, L.I., Watts, D.T., and Howell, T. The Doctor-Nurse Game Revisited. *New England J Med* 322:546-549, 1990.
15. Pence, T. &, Cantrall, I. *Ethics In Nursing: An Anthology.* Chapter 6, The Nurse-Physician Relationship: Whistleblowing. pp. 215-217.
16. Curtin, L. Nurses and Physicians: Of Gnats and Humbugs. *Curtin Calls,* West Dundee, IL, S-N Publications, 1989, pp. 61-63.
17. Commonwealth of Pennsylvania: Professional Nursing Law. P.L. 432, No. 151, 1986.

18. Commonwealth of Pennsylvania: Legal Code (143338) § 186 May 1990, pp. 21-80.
19. Nightingale, F. "Sick Nursing and Health Nursing." In Isabel A. Hamton, et al., *Nursing of the Sick 1893.* New York, McGraw-Hill, 1949, pp. 24-25.
20. Meyer, R.H., Mannix, M.N., and Costello, T.F. Nursing Recruitment: Do Health Care Managers Gear Strategies to the Appropriate Audience? *Hosp Hlth Serv Admin* 36: 447-453, 1991.
21. Alt, J.M., and Houston, G.R. (Eds.). *Nursing Career Ladders; A Practical Manual.* Rockville, MD, Aspen, 1986.
22. Weinstein, G.W. Professional Dissonance: Balancing personal imperfection and professional genius. *Bull Am Coll Surg* 76: 19, 1991.
23. I should like to thank: Professor Elaine Larson, Johns Hopkins University School of Nursing; and from the Guthrie Health Care System, Dr. Kenneth K. Meyer F.A.C.S., Ms. Carolyn Corbett, R.N., M.S., Ms. Jean Antes, M.A., M.L.S., for their critical reviews and invaluable suggestions.

The Heroic Physician in Literature: Can The Tradition Continue?*

Anne Hudson Jones

Anne Hudson Jones is Professor of Literature and Medicine in the Institute for the Medical Humanities at The University of Texas Medical Branch, Galveston, Texas. Before joining the Institute faculty in 1979, she was Assistant Director of the Center for Programs in the Humanities at Virginia Polytechnic Institute and State University in Blacksburg, Virginia. She received her Ph.D. in Comparative Literature from the University of North Carolina at Chapel Hill in 1974.

One of the founding editors of *Literature and Medicine,* Professor Jones served as the journal's Editor-in-Chief for ten years (1984-1993). At the request of the Editorial Board, she has continued her association with the journal as Senior Consulting Editor. In addition to several special issues of the journal that she has edited—*Images of Healers (*1983), *Tenth Anniversary Retrospective* (1991), *General Issue* (1992), *General Issue* (1993), and *Science Fiction and the Future of Medicine* (2001)—she is the editor of *Images of Nurses: Perspectives from History, Art, and Literature* (University of Pennsylvania Press, 1988; Japanese translation, 1997), and co-editor with Faith McLellan of *Ethical Issues in Biomedical Publication* (Johns Hopkins University Press, 2000). She has also published numerous articles, chapters, and reviews about various aspects of literature and medicine, including a well-received series in *The Lancet.*

In 1991, Dr. Jones received the President's Award of the American Medical Writers Association, and in 2003 she received the Nicholas E. Davies Memorial Scholar Award of the American College of Physicians.

*Delivered 12 May 1993 at the Twenty-third Annual Meeting of the American Osler Society, Louisville, Kentucky

In the 1938 Hollywood film *Young Dr. Kildare,* the second of sixteen movies in this popular series, Jimmy Kildare explains to his childhood sweetheart why he can't stay in Dartford, Connecticut, and go into practice with his father, a country doctor. He says,

> There [are] two ways of being a doctor: One is for the living you can make out of it. Now I could marry you and settle down and count on taking over my father's practice. . . . [But] being a doctor can be bigger than three meals a day. Ehrlich was that kind of a doctor; so was Lister. I'm certainly no Lister, but . . .[1]

Young Dr. Kildare does not yet know exactly what kind of doctor he wants to be, but he does know that he is not in medicine only for the living he can make from it. He has been inspired by the heroic tradition of doctors such as Ehrlich and Lister to seek something more. Sir William Osler was also the kind of physician who inspired, and continues to inspire, other physicians to practice medicine as a special profession, almost as a secular holy calling. The existence of the American Osler Society attests to the continuing power of the heroic tradition in medicine. It is the development and decline of this tradition as it is reflected in literature that is my subject here.

The heroic tradition of medicine and doctors does not have a long history in literature. By contrast, the comic tradition of physicians in literature goes back many centuries. In Western culture, writers have always made fun of doctors. An oft-quoted biblical injunction sets the tone: "He that sinneth before his Maker, let him fall into the hands of the physicians."[2] By the Middle Ages, the physician appeared in literature as a stock character, ridiculed or portrayed as a quack. Examples include the physicians in Boccaccio's *Decameron* (ca. 1351), Chaucer's *Canterbury Tales* (1387-1400), and the Italian *commedia dell'art.* This comic tradition of stupid, greedy physician-quacks reached its peak in Molière's comedies in seventeenth-century France: *Le Médecin volant (The Flying Doctor), Dom Juan (Don Juan), ¼ Amour médecin (Doctor Cupid), Le Médecin malgré lui (The Doctor in Spite of Himself),* and *Le Malade imaginaire (The Imaginary Invalid),* all written and first performed between 1658 and 1673. It was not until the nineteenth century that the physician in literature took on heroic characteristics. The temporal correlation between the appearance of the heroic physician in literature and the development of medical science is no coincidence. Only when medicine had begun to develop as a modern empirical science that might eventually be able to offer efficacious treatments for patients did the physician in literature acquire the attributes of a hero.

The heroic physician as a character type begins to appear in Western literature around the mid-nineteenth century (just about the time of Osler's birth in

1849), reaches its peak in the 1930s and 1940s (a decade or two after Osler's death in 1919), and is in decline by the 1970s. Thus, in the second half of the nineteenth century and the first half of the twentieth, many works of the Western literary canon featured heroic physicians. Some of the best-known examples are Gustave Flaubert's *Madame Bovary* (1857); George Eliot's *Middlemarch* (1871-1872); Ibsen's *An Enemy of the People* (1882); Émile Zola's *Docteur Pascal* (1893); Sinclair Lewis's *Arrowsmith* (1925); Sidney Howard's *Yellow Jack* (1933); Sidney Kingsley's *Men in White* (1933); A. J. Cronin's *The Citadel* (1937); and Albert Camus's *The Plague* (1947). I will use four of these works—*Madame Bovary*, *Middlemarch*, *Arrowsmith*, and *The Plague*—to outline briefly the development of this tradition and to establish the heroic attributes of its physician characters. Embedded within their heroic attributes are the very qualities that have led to the decline of this tradition in contemporary literature.

Flaubert's *Madame Bovary* (1857), subtitled *A Story of Provincial Life*, may seem an odd choice for first mention in discussion of this tradition of heroic physicians in literature. Certainly there is nothing heroic about Charles Bovary, who is characterized early in the novel as being "like a mill-horse tramping round blindfold, grinding away at he knows not what" (p. 22).[3] Bovary is a fool, set at the study of medicine not out of any sense of calling but because his father is an ex-assistant-surgeon-major. Indeed, Bovary has no heroic aspirations nor any greater expectations of medicine than that it provide him a reasonable living. Presented with "lectures on anatomy, lectures on pathology, lectures on physiology, lectures on pharmacy, on chemistry and botany, on diagnosis and therapy, not to mention hygiene and materia medica," he "didn't understand a word of it; couldn't grasp it . . ." (p. 22). After failing his exams once, he manages to memorize the questions and pass the next time. But he is licensed only as an Officer of Health—not as a full-fledged physician. Although Bovary can set uncomplicated leg fractures and deal with other straightforward medical problems, he cannot successfully carry out more complicated or innovative treatments. Yet his wife and the local pharmacist persuade him, against his better judgment—feeble as it is—to try a new surgical treatment for strephopodia (clubfoot) on the Yonville stable boy, Hippolyte. Although the operation is reported in the local newspaper as a success, Hippolyte develops gangrene and must have his leg amputated.

No, Charles Bovary does not exemplify characteristics of the heroic physician. He is more like the stock character of the physician-quack, set now in a realistic rather than a comic context. His failures, however, provide occasions for a glimpse of two successively more heroic-appearing physicians. The fifty-year-old Dr. Canivet—a bona fide Doctor of Medicine—is summoned from Neufchatel to amputate Hippolyte's leg and thereby save his life. Dr. Canivet makes no secret of his scorn for Bovary, one of those Officers of Health who degrade the profession of medicine that Canivet considers a sacred calling. Yet Canivet is equally contemptuous of the specialists in Paris who would even dream of straightening a clubfoot. Canivet represents limited medical competence without heroic aspirations; he is content with his present knowledge and sees nothing good to come from efforts to extend the realm of medical knowledge and treatment. Next to Bovary, Canivet looks heroic simply because he is more competent in Hippolyte's case.

Dr. Canivet's measure is taken again, however, near the end of the novel, when he is called to attend Madame Bovary, who has poisoned herself with arsenic. Shortly after Canivet arrives and prescribes an emetic, the great Dr. Larivière arrives from Paris. His arrival is compared to that of a god, and he is described as one of those "who cherished their art with a fanatical love and practised it with zeal and sagacity" (p. 331). Larivière, disdainful of honors, titles, and decorations, is characterized as an intellectual, a truth seeker, who "might almost have passed for a saint had not his mental acuity caused him to be feared as a demon" (p. 331). He belongs to "that great line of surgeons that sprang from Bichat [1771-1802]" (p. 331). In private, Larivière rebukes Canivet for having given the emetic. No longer the arrogant physician railing about Officers of Health, Canivet has been put in his place by a greater physician, one he dares not contradict. Next to Larivière, Canivet looks decidedly unheroic—not even competent in Madame Bovary's case.

Larivière's attributes recur, in differing combinations, in later heroic physicians in literature. Foremost among these attributes are great talent, a keen intellect employed in the rigorous search for truth, and a savage disregard for material rewards and earthly honors. One more—compassion—bears mention: Confronted with the death agony of Madame Bovary, whom he has arrived too late to save, Lariviere sheds a tear that drops onto his shirt. Despite his years of experience with such scenes, he is still moved by Emma Bovary's suffering and by Charles Bovary's grief.

Flaubert's Larivière, a *deus ex machina* come too late, is only a minor character in *Madame Bovary,* but he foreshadows the heroic physicians soon to come. In *Middlemarch* (1871-1872), the first great English novel to present a physician as its hero, George Eliot characterizes Tertius Lydgate in much greater depth. Lydgate's "moment of vocation" comes when, as a young boy, he opens the encyclopedia and begins reading under the heading "Anatomy": "From that hour Lydgate felt the growth of an intellectual passion" (p. 98).[4] He studies in London, Edinburgh, and Paris, and believes that "the medical profession as it might be was the finest in the world; presenting the most perfect interchange between science and art; offering the most direct alliance between intellectual conquest and the social good" (p. 99). He wants both to reform medicine and to "work out the proof of an anatomical conception and make a link in the chain of discovery" (p. 100). In the year 1829, when Lydgate goes into practice in Middlemarch, "the dark territories of Pathology were a fine America for a spirited young adventurer" (p. 101). Lydgate wants to combine the practice of medicine and surgery, reform the profession of medicine, "contribute towards enlarging the scientific, rational basis of his profession"

(p. 101), and carry on Bichat's work by discovering "the primitive tissue" (p. 102); in short, he wants "to do good small work for Middlemarch, and great work for the world" (p. 102).

Flaubert tells nothing of Larivière's personal life, but Eliot tells much about Lydgate's. Lydgate meets and impulsively marries Rosamond Vincy, the prettiest woman in town. She has no understanding of Lydgate's true love of medicine as calling and expects him to pursue it only for the successful living it will provide her. Osler has this to say about Lydgate: "This well-drawn character in George Eliot's 'Middlemarch' may be studied with advantage by the physician; one of the most important lessons to be gathered from it is—marry the right woman."[5] I do not dispute this. But the larger point is that keen intelligence and great competence in the scientific and technical aspects of medicine are necessary but not sufficient for the truly heroic physician to achieve his goals; he must exercise self-discipline and mature judgment in personal as well as professional matters, lest he ruin his "intellectual life in a soul-wasting struggle with worldly annoyances," as Osler puts it.[6] The fault, however, is Lydgate's, not Rosamond's. As Eliot phrases it, Lydgate's heroic character is flawed by "spots of commonness": that is, "that distinction of mind which belonged to his intellectual ardour, did not penetrate his feeling and judgment about furniture, or women, or the desirability of its being known (without his telling) that he was better born than other country surgeons" (p. 103). Although he wants to be one of the great men of medicine, he expects to have all the accouterments of a comfortable life. After he fails in Middlemarch and moves to London, he sets up a highly successful practice among the wealthy and becomes "what is called a successful man" (p. 575). Yet he regards himself a failure because "he had not done what he once meant to do" (p. 575). He dies prematurely, of diphtheria, leaving Rosamond and his children well provided for by a heavy insurance on his life, but leaving his profession unreformed and the primitive tissue undiscovered. Lydgate has heroic attributes and aspirations but because of his "spots of commonness"—his tragic flaw, if you will—he never fulfills his potential.

Appearing half a century after *Middlemarch,* Sinclair Lewis's *Arrowsmith* (1925), the preeminent American novel about a heroic physician, develops and extends this tradition in literature. Like Lydgate, Martin Arrowsmith receives his call to medicine as a profession when he is a young boy, in his case by reading *Gray's Anatomy* and helping old Doc Vickerson, an alcoholic, in his rather questionable practice of medicine. Instead of being educated in London, Edinburgh, and Paris, however, Arrowsmith attends the fictional University of Winnemac, a large Midwestern state university, probably based on the University of Michigan. In the medical school there, he is inspired by two quite different physicians: Max Gottlieb, a German, Jewish professor of bacteriology, who has worked with Koch and Pasteur and represents for Arrowsmith the ideal of scientific research; and T. J. H. "Dad" Silva, professor of internal medicine and dean of the medical school, who represents the Oslerian ideal of clinical medicine, as Lewis makes clear—"Silva's god was Sir William Osler, his religion was the art of sympathetic healing, and his patriotism was accurate physical diagnosis" (p. 82)[7] Arrowsmith initially gives up research for marriage to Leora Tozer and starts a private practice in Leora's hometown, Wheatsylvania, North Dakota. Unlike Lydgate, Arrowsmith has married the right kind of wife—this time, anyway. Leora loves him completely, sacrifices her life to his, and wants nothing more. The thing Arrowsmith likes most about her is "her singular ability to be cheerfully non-existent even when she [is] present" (p. 324). As Gottlieb has predicted, however, Arrowsmith fails at private practice and later fails at public health work. Arrowsmith is no "Dad" Silva. When he is finally given the opportunity to join Gottlieb at the McGurk Institute in New York City, Arrowsmith finds his true vocation: not medical practice, but scientific research. Gottlieb tells him he has the qualities necessary in a scientist: he is curious and stubborn, and he does not accept rules. Gottlieb then contrasts the true scientist with the ordinary man:

> To be a scientist—it is not just a different job, so that a man should choose between being a scientist and being an explorer or abond-salesman or a physician or a king or a farmer. . . . [I]t makes its victim all different from the good normal man. The normal man, he does not care much what he does except that he should eat and sleep and make love. But the scientist is intensely religious—he is so religious that he will not accept quarter-truths, because they are an insult to his faith.
>
> . . . He [the scientist] speaks no meaner of the ridiculous faith-healers and chiropractors than he does of the doctors that want to snatch our science before it is tested and rush around hoping they heal people, and spoiling all the clues with their footsteps. . . . (p. 267)

Gottlieb closes this exhortation by telling Arrowsmith that to be a scientist is born in a man and that he will do his best to protect Arrowsmith from that American bitch-goddess Success, the destroyer of good science—and good scientists. He concludes: "May Koch bless you!" (p. 268).

In this famous scene, Gottlieb portrays the attributes of the practicing physician—the Silvas inspired by Osler—as inferior to those of the scientist. Silva's religion of sympathetic healing is scorned by Gottlieb in his praise of the religion of science. And at this point in Western literature, the heroic physician is displaced by the heroic physician-scientist, with the emphasis on scientist. The sympathetic physician may do some "good small work," but it is the scientist who will do "great work for the world" *(Middlemarch,* p. 102*)*. In Lewis's novel no one—physician or scientist—is portrayed as able to do both. Lydgate's ideal of combining them is no longer feasible; Arrowsmith must choose between them.

Arrowsmith's big chance comes when he is sent to a plague-infested island in the West Indies to carry out an experiment on the efficacy of an antiplague phage. Gottlieb rigorously instructs Arrowsmith to give the phage to half the residents and deny it to the other half. True to his mentor, Arrowsmith tries to carry out the controlled experiment. But after his wife, Leora, dies of plague, Arrowsmith, in his grief, gives the phage to all who want it. When he returns to New York to confess his failure, he finds that he has lost Gottlieb to senile dementia. Ironically, despite his failure, Arrowsmith is given a hero's welcome in New York, is soon remarried—this time to a beautiful woman of wealth and considerable social position—and then is offered the assistant directorship of the McGurk Institute, with the expectation that he would become the director of the Institute within two years. He declines the offer, abandons his new wife and son, and runs away to the Vermont woods with one of his true-scientist buddies. The novel ends with Arrowsmith's words: "I feel as if I were really beginning to work now. . . . We'll plug along . . . for two or three years, and maybe we'll get something permanent—and probably we'll fail!" (p. 430). Arrowsmith breaks free of the bonds of marriage and society that imprison Lydgate; he accepts external failure as the price of true personal success in doing good science; and he understands that the quest is its own reward. Thus, he is portrayed as more heroic than Lydgate. But Arrowsmith is heroic only as a scientist, not as a physician.

Just as *Madame Bovary* is a pivotal work, looking both backward and forward in its characterizations of physicians, so is Albert Camus's novel *The Plague* (1947). Its protagonist, Dr. Rieux, is heroic because of circumstance: he practices medicine in a passionate effort to fight relentlessly against death, even though in time of plague he cannot win. For Camus, Rieux is an absurd hero, trying to do the impossible, knowing it is impossible. Because he is battling an ancient disease with no effective weapon, Rieux is like physicians from past eras. He is the model for the image that William F. May identifies as the physician as fighter.[8] Because he cannot succeed, Rieux is free to try with all his might. His is a world of plague, failure, and death, but it is a simple world: it is clear what is evil, and it is clear that evil should be opposed. The allegorical aspects of this novel—the plague representing the Nazi occupation of France in World War II—help explain this simplicity. In the early years of the AIDS epidemic, before anyone understood what was really happening and while people were referring to the mysterious disease as a plague, many of the articles and books about AIDS used epigraphs from Camus's *The Plague.* In the face of such a killer disease, resistance seemed the only humane or heroic response. Dr. Rieux and his plague fighters, most of them ordinary men who accept their responsibility to work and fight for the communal good, provided a compelling image of heroism for those who struggled against AIDS with no effective weapon.

Dr. Rieux is not a researcher. He has a modest private practice and no dreams of contributing to the history of medical science and discovery. His heroism comes from his self-sacrificing devotion to medicine and from his stalwartness throughout the plague. Rieux seems more intelligent and honest than most of the others in the city of Oran, but he insists that he is no more heroic than others: "there's no question of heroism in all this," he says. "It's a matter of common decency."[9] He does what he can do. In his unremitting fight against death, he looks backward to prescientific physicians who were impotent in the face of disease and death; yet he also foreshadows the image of the modern physician as unheroic technician.

In summary, the heroic physicians in these novels are all white men, of European or Anglo extraction; they are "called" to the profession of medicine or medical science; they have extraordinary intelligence and talent; their profession becomes a replacement religion or philosophy for them; they practice it to do more than just make a living from it; they care more about intellectual knowledge and truth than they care about success in material or worldly terms; and to be successful they must sacrifice personal and family relationships to their work. These characteristics sound lofty, idealistic, truly heroic. Why, then, might such a tradition be in danger or decline?

This tradition is currently challenged by many different medical and cultural changes. I will focus on four: first, the remarkable success of medical technology in keeping bodies alive indefinitely (with the concomitant high costs); second, the continuing impotence of medicine to cure many diseases—represented most powerfully by AIDS; third, the social changes in gender roles; and, fourth, the assault on Western values by an increasingly multicultural population.

The first two of these challenges are clearly reflected in British and American literature of the 1970s and 1980s. An interesting shift has taken place, with the patient displacing the physician as hero, especially in drama. Mel Gussow, the *New York Times* drama critic, wrote about this shift in 1979 in an article titled "The Time of the Wounded Hero."[10] In 1979, AIDS was still unknown; Gussow was writing about plays such as Michael Cristofer's *The Shadow Box* (1977), Arthur Kopit's *Wings* (1978), Brian Clark's *Whose Life Is It Anyway?* (1978), and Bernard Pomerance's *Elephant Man* (1979). As I have written elsewhere, part of what seems to have been going on was that " [t]o the age-old fear of suffering serious injury or illness, we now have added the peculiarly contemporary fear of becoming a victim of sophisticated medical technology, whose 'miracles' can prolong the impaired lives and suffering of people, sometimes against their will."[11] Also, developing out of the civil rights movement, the women's movement, and a growing distrust of professionals, the patients' rights movement had come of age. In many ways, this movement was a response to the physician as unheroic technician. May's discussion helps explain how the heroic physician-fighter Dr. Rieux leads to the unheroic physician-technician:

> The spectacular success of modern medical technology has reinforced

> the definition of the physician as fighter. It creates a cultural momentum; it produces a moral scheme out of the technologist's impulse: what can be done should be done. . . . [I]n recent times, a piety toward the machine argues for the endless prolongation of life. The sheer existence of the machinery and a team that knows how to use it argues for its mechanical employment. The machine becomes autonomous. Instead of the machine saving the patient's life and assisting that person's recovery so as to permit him or her once again to serve others, the patient serves the machine.[12]

No more devastating literary example of this tendency can be found than Kurt Vonnegut's story "Fortitude" (1968), in which a hundred-year-old woman has become only a head on a tripod connected to a mass of pipes and tubing.[13] She begs to die, but her physician, Dr. Norbert Frankenstein, is caught up in a technological creative frenzy, proudest of the artificial pancreas that cost as much as the State of Vermont. The Westinghouse artificial heart he dismisses as merely a sixty-thousand-dollar pump. The patient, Sylvia Lovejoy, begs her beautician to help her, and the beautician brings her a gun. But Sylvia's prosthetic arms have been designed so that she cannot point a gun at herself or get poison to her lips. When Sylvia discovers this as she tries to shoot herself, she turns the gun toward Dr. Frankenstein and shoots him instead. The ironic twist, however, is that Dr. Frankenstein has designed all the artificial organs so that they can sustain two bodies, not just one. He has himself hooked up next to Sylvia, and the two of them are together—presumably for eternity. Vonnegut parodies current medical and cultural practices to dramatize the need to set limits somewhere, to pull the plug when a human being has become an assemblage of artificial parts. Further, Vonnegut shows the impulse toward this kind of horrific immortality coming just as much, if not more so, from technologically impelled physicians as from patients.

Another literary perspective on this kind of technological medicine gone awry comes from Samuel Shem's infamous *The House of God* (1978). In this novel, physicians are extremely competent medical technicians who can keep patients alive long after they wish to be dead. The demented old people who are not allowed to die—the so called gomers, human beings who have "lost—often through age—what goes into being a human being" (p. 424)—are perhaps the best-known examples.[14] But the death of the Man with Agonal Respirations shows contemporary medicine's difficulty in letting a young person—even when comatose and terminally ill with end-stage multiple myeloma and renal failure—die in peace. When the Man with Agonal Respirations tries to die, he is resuscitated, transferred to the Medical Intensive Care Unit, and hooked up to a respirator. Medicine as practiced in this novel makes no human sense; its technology terrorizes patients as well as any doctors who still manage to care about their patients as persons. Performing technological miracles Charles Bovary and Canivet could never have dreamed of, these physicians have much in common with the blindfolded mill-horse, "grinding away at he knows not what" (*Madame Bovary,* p. 22).

I want to mention one more literary example from the 1970s: Brian Clark's drama *Whose Life Is It Anyway?* (1978). In this work, which played successfully in London and New York and was eventually made into a movie, a young sculptor has become a quadriplegic as the result of an automobile accident. The doctors have saved his life, stabilized him, and now plan to ship him out to a nursing home or long-term care facility. When the patient, Ken Harrison, asks that treatment be withheld so that he can die, the consultant physician, Dr. Michael Emerson, has a psychiatrist diagnose Harrison as clinically depressed and therefore unable to make a rational decision. Dr. Emerson continues to treat Harrison against his wishes. Harrison retains legal counsel, gets a hearing, and wins his right to have treatment discontinued. The response to this play—which was surprisingly popular given its depressing subject matter—demonstrated a widespread public interest in patients' rights to determine the course of their own treatment rather than be the recipient of medical paternalism's sense of beneficence. It is worth noting that the younger physician in this play, a woman named Clare Scott, is at odds with Emerson, her chief, over his continued treatment of Harrison. She listens to Harrison and is personally and professionally troubled by his plight. Although her gender may have nothing to do with her response, there are so few women physicians depicted in literature that her gender cannot be disregarded.

These three—"Fortitude," *The House of God*, and *Whose Life Is It Anyway?*—are representative of many contemporary literary works that take medicine as their subject. Ironically, the physician-scientist has been so successful in his work that the presumed beneficiaries of that work are rebelling against it; scientific discovery has given way to technological imperative, which seems devoid of any values other than technical competence for its own sake. The mill-horse keeps making his rounds.

The second challenge to the tradition is, on the face of it, the complete opposite of technological prowess: it is medicine's impotence. By the mid-1980s, literature began to reflect yet another medical and cultural crisis—AIDS. The complacent assumption that infectious diseases were eradicated, or at least under control, at least in first-world countries, gave way to reports of a strange new virus against which medical science seemed completely helpless. In the early days of the AIDS epidemic, allegedly because of the groups first infected, there was not the heroic medical and scientific response many hoped for.

In the early literature about AIDS, especially the AIDS plays, as they have become known—Larry Kramer's *The Normal Heart* (1985), William Hoffman's *As Is* (1985), and Harvey Fierstein's *Safe Sex* (1987)—doctors and nurses are barely there. Dr. Emma Brookner of *The Normal Heart* is an exception: female, German but often mistaken for Jewish, in a wheelchair because she is a survivor of polio, she cares for more gay men in New York City than does any other practitioner, but she cannot get a grant to fund her research on these patients. Kramer based Brookner's character on Dr. Linda Laubenstein, "the wheelchair-bound pioneer of AIDS work in New York City."[15] Alluded to in many of the literary works about AIDS is the feud between the American and the French researchers over who first discovered the AIDS virus. Instead of looking heroic, the researchers represented in these works look as if they are primarily concerned with their own fame and glory.

But the AIDS plays are by no means the first works of contemporary literature to show the helplessness of medicine to heal or the failure of physicians to care for those patients they cannot cure. Peter Nichols's *Joe Egg* (1967) and Marsha Norman's *'night, Mother* (1983) are two well-known examples. *Joe Egg* is the story of the young couple Bri and Sheila, who are trying to care for their multiply handicapped daughter—"a kind of living parsnip," as Sheila calls her.[16] They receive no support—moral or otherwise—from the physicians they consult about their daughter's condition and care. In *'night, Mother,* a young woman commits suicide because her epilepsy has made life seem to her not worth living. Medicine has offered nothing that helps her deal with the anguish of her condition.

The point here is not just that medicine is impotent to cure AIDS, epilepsy, and congenital handicaps, but that many people receive no comfort or caring from their physicians. Medicine offers these patients neither cure nor comfort. The sense that physicians are professionally detached and personally unmoved by their suffering sparks bitterness in patients—and results in satirical images of physicians in literature.

The third challenge to this tradition of heroic male physicians comes from changing gender roles. Women have entered medical schools in ever increasing numbers during the 1970s and 1980s. And as women have come into medicine, they have inevitably brought some of their own perspectives and values with them. They are not likely to find husbands who will subordinate themselves so totally as Leora Arrowsmith did to a physician-spouse's career. Yet most of these young women hope to marry and have families. There are not many literary works about women physicians, but the few I know from the late nineteenth century make it clear that a woman who wants to be a physician must give up any ideas of having a family. Twentieth-century works have not challenged that assumption until very recently, probably because there have not yet been many women physician-writers.

For a quick glimpse of the gender and cultural differences that contemporary women physicians struggle with, I know of nowhere better to turn than Perri Klass's "Baby Poop" (1987). In this short essay, Klass describes her conflicting maternal and medical responses as she, as a medical student, accompanies the neurology consult team to see a baby in the newborn nursery. An unmistakable odor from the bassinet announces the baby's need to have his diaper changed. Klass, herself the mother of a small child, volunteers to change the diaper. All the doctors tell her not to: they will do their exam; then the nurse can change the diaper. The neurological exam takes almost an hour; the physicians ignore their own discomfort, as well as the baby's. The situation leads Klass to reflect on "various kinds of arrogance."[17]

The fourth challenge to this heroic tradition comes from demographic changes in the United States (and elsewhere) that are creating a more multicultural population than ever before. More and more physicians practicing in this country are of African, Hispanic, Asian, Indian, or Arabic ethnicity. These physicians may not share the values of the Anglo-European tradition that are reflected in Western medicine and in works of the Western literary canon. For example, they may not place the high value on individualism and autonomy that Western culture does. In the scene from *The House of God* in which the code has been called for the Man with Agonal Respirations, Shem describes the Hindu anesthesiologist, who "pumped oxygen at the head of the bed, looking over the mess with a compassionate disdain, perhaps thinking back to the dead beggars littering dawn in Bombay" (*House of God,* p. 286). The effort and resources expended to prolong the life of a single dying person in this country must look very strange to someone from an economically poorer country.

Ironically, in a time when medical miracles are commonplace, physicians in literature are oddly unheroic. The heroic tradition has been displaced by satire, more bitter now than it was in the earlier comic tradition. Can the tradition of the heroic physician in literature continue? All I can offer are my speculations: if the tradition survives, it will do so because it has responded to these contemporary challenges in ways that revitalize and transform the heroic paradigm. Some aspects will remain the same, I believe. Heroic physicians in literature will continue to have great intelligence and talent, and they will go into medicine because they perceive it as a special calling. Other features, I predict, will change: First, heroic physicians will no longer all be men of Anglo or European extraction. There will be women among them—and men and women of every race and ethnicity. Second, heroic physicians will no longer sacrifice their personal and family relationships so totally to their work. They will place more value on such relationships and will struggle to balance love and work. Third, for these future heroic physicians, the values of science will be subordinated to human values. And, finally, the heroic quest will no longer require exploration of new frontiers—geographic or scientific; instead, the quest will be to live and practice within limits, to rein in technology and make it serve the communal human good. Larivière provides a helpful model here. When he cannot relieve suffering or prevent death, he allows himself to feel and express his compassion. Neither his limits nor his tears lessen his heroic stature. Rather, they affirm it.

Medicine is not alone in facing these challenges, but as a compelling microcosm of society at large, it offers an arena in which conflicts of cultural and moral values are dramatically displayed. And literary images are not exact reflections of reality, of course, even in works of literary Realism. Yet there is an integral relationship between what is happening in medicine and the way medicine and physicians are represented in literature. In times of such major cultural changes, what real physicians do as they practice their profession has potential consequences that go beyond the immediate moment and the individual patient.

As I prepared this lecture, I thought a lot about what Osler might say in regard to these matters. I believe that were he still alive, he would be in the forefront of those leading the constructive response of medicine to these contemporary challenges.

References

1. From *Young Dr. Kildare,* MGM, 1938. This was the first of the *Dr. Kildare* films to feature the famous cast of Lew Ayres, as Dr. Jimmy Kildare, and Lionel Barrymore, as Dr. Leonard Gillespie.
2. Ecclesiasticus 38:15, from the Apocrypha. Kathryn Montgomery Hunter quotes this verse in the opening paragraph of her article "The Satiric Image, Healers in *The House of God,*" *Literature and Medicine* 2:135, 1983; and Richard Reynolds and John Stone include an excerpt from Ecclesiasticus 38 in their anthology of literature for medical students, *On Doctoring, Stories: Poems, Essays.* New York, Simon and Schuster, 1991, p. 23. Unfortunately, a typographical error in *On Doctoring* changes the meaning of the verse completely: "He who *sings* before his Maker, may he fall into the care of a physician." [My italics.]
3. Gustave Flaubert. *Madame Bovary: A Story of Provincial Life* (1857), trans. Alan Russell. Baltimore, Penguin Books, 1965. All quotations from the novel are from this translation and are cited parenthetically in my text.
4. George Eliot. *Middlemarch* (1871-72), Bert G. Homback, (Ed.). Critical Edition, New York. Norton, 1977. All quotations from the novel are from this edition and are cited parenthetically in my text.
5. Sir William Osler, quoted in Harvey Cushing, *The Life of Sir William Osler,* 3d impression, vol. 1. Oxford, Clarendon Press, 1925, pp. 462-63.
6. Ibid., p. 463, n. 1.
7. Sinclair Lewis. *Arrowsmith.* New York, New American Library, Signet Classic, 1925. All quotations from the novel are from this edition and are cited parenthetically in my text.
8. William F. May. *The Physician's Covenant, Images of the Healer in Medical Ethics.* Philadelphia, Westminister Press, 1983, pp. 63-86.
9. Albert Camus. *The Plague* (1947), trans. Stuart Gilbert. New York, Modern Library, 1948, p. 150.
10. Mel Gussow. "The Time of the Wounded Healer," *New York Times,* 15 April 1979, sec. 2, pp. 1, 30.
11. Anne Hudson Jones. "Literature and Medicine: Illness from the Patient's

Point of View," in *Personal Choices and Public Commitments: Perspectives on the Medical Humanities,* William J. Winslade (Ed.) Galveston, TX, Institute for the Medical Humanities, 1988, p. 1.
12. May, pp. 64-65.
13. Kurt Vonnegut, Jr. "Fortitude" (1968), in *Human-Machines: An Anthology of Stories about Cyborgs*, T.N. Scortia and G. Zebrowski (Eds.). New York Random House, Vintage Books, 1975, pp. 39-59. "Fortitude" originally appeared in *Playboy*.
14. Samuel Shem. *The House of God* (1978), 10th anniversary ed. New York, Dell, 1988. All quotations from the novel are from this edition and are cited parenthetically in my text.
15. Randy Shilts. *And the Band Played On: Politics, People, and the AIDS Epidemic* New York, St. Martin's, 1987, p. 531.
16. Peter Nichols. *Joe Egg.* New York, Grove Press, 1967.
17. Perri Klass. "Baby Poop," in *A Not Entirely Benign Procedure: Four Years as a Medical Student.* New York, G. P. Putnam's Sons, 1987, p. 166.

"The Leaven of Science": Osler and Medical Research*

David Hamilton

David Hamilton trained in transplant surgery at the Western Infirmary, Glasgow, and studied immunology under Sir Peter Medawar in London. He later spent time at the Wellcome Unit for the History of Medicine at Oxford, before returning as a surgeon to Glasgow.

In addition to his numerous scientific publications, he is author of *The Healers, A History of Medicine in Scotland* (1981), and *The Monkey Gland Affair* (1983) an account of testis transplantation in the 1920s. He is a book collector, and in addition to his holdings relevant to Scottish medicine and surgery, he has a large library of books on golf and his *Golf–Scotland's Game* (1998) is a standard reference work.

Since 1984 Mr. Hamilton has run his own private press—The Partick Press—which uses traditional letterpress printing on fine mould-made paper. Under this imprint he prints and publishes his own writings on the history of golf in Scotland.

---

*Delivered 10 May 1994 at the Twenty-fourth Annual Meeting of the American Osler Society, London and Oxford, England

When we survey William Osler's remarkable abilities and acknowledge his skills as a clinician, author, teacher, historian, bibliophile and bibliographer there is however a moment's delay in adding 'researcher' to this list. But after this hesitation, we immediately recall his considerable list of publications, and his time in the pathology laboratory, a place which at that time, was the powerhouse for medical innovation. Infectious disease was then dominant, as the headings for his textbook show, and the pathology/bacteriology laboratory was the center of research. His personal studies were rewarded by having left behind at least two eponymous diseases, and claims to a third.

Nor should we look to Osler or his contemporaries for any advance in therapeutics. His was a time of therapeutic stagnation. He himself pronounced that only iodine, iron, mercury, quinine, and digitalis were essential medications, adding cocaine later. There was little movement in the pharmacopoeia in his lifetime. It was still enough to be a naturalist, an observer of the experiments of nature, and Osler did this characteristically well. Perhaps it was his conviction that a man's best research days are over by the age of forty, and his own pursuit of other matters thereafter, that make us forget his involvement when young in the pursuit of medical progress.

But there remains a nagging doubt. Here and there in his works, Osler expresses some reservations about the role of medical research. What I would suggest to you to resolve this paradox is that while Osler did everything in his power to assist the progress of medicine, it was his view that there were limits to the role of research in the larger world. His view, I think, was that the doctor's life's work was not one to be dominated by research, nor did he approve of some of those who permitted this. Research was to be a 'leaven'—an addition introduced into the mix of medical practice—but only needed in small quantities, and certainly not to be taken on its own.

Osler and Research

I propose to examine Osler's support of medical research. I will deal in detail with his period in Oxford from 1908, after leaving Hopkins, until his death in 1919. This will fit with your Society's visit to England, and may illuminate, even for the most ardent students of Osler's career, some less well-known facets. There has been recent scholarly interest in the early support of medical research in the London hospitals, notably studies of the early academic teaching units in London, and in the early days of MRC - the British Medical Research Council, our equivalent of the National Institutes of Health. It is fascinating to discover Osler's role in these events, a part played fairly inconspicuously, but as you will see, a vital one.

Let us first demonstrate his commitment of medical research. It is easily done. During a visit to Germany, he saw what was possible, and he wrote to

August Hoch back at Hopkins in 1890.

> The presence in every [German] medical center of a class of men devoted to scientific work gives a totally different aspect to professional aspirations. While with us—and in England—the young man may start with an ardent desire to devote his life to science, he is soon dragged into the mill of practice, and at forty years of age 'the guinea stamp' is on all his work . . . we sadly miss the leaven which such a class would bring into our professional life.[1]

This total commitment to medical science is striking, as is his apparent support of the full-time system, a controversy to which we will return. We can now follow Osler's links with medical science while in England.

Osler came to Oxford in 1905. At one level he declared that his great wish in life was to be close to the great libraries in Britain and to have *The [London] Times* on his breakfast table each morning. His first years were spent in pleasant uninvolvement with wider matters. He continued to collect and buy and visit bookshops and dealers. There were many pleasant chores—lectures to British Medical Association branches, worthy prize-givings, social visits to social gatherings such as the Cowes regatta, and jaunts to the Scottish Highlands to the castle of the Lovats at Inverness. Even public issues seemed ephemeral—he was involved briefly with a Royal Commission into the use of vivisection in research, but the antivivisectionist lobby failed to change established practice much and the matter dropped from public view.

New Challenges

But thereafter Osler slowly became drawn into the public events of the time. Close to home, the Oxford University Press had, surprisingly, no medical book list. Osler as a Regent to the Press encouraged such projects, and soon he and they had started what was to be one of the world's great medical journals—*The Quarterly Journal of Medicine.*

Another important issue of the time was dissatisfaction with health care in Britain. There was concern about the level of health of the ordinary people, not unconnected with the Boer War and the military defeat in South Africa, where the average British soldier was much inferior in physique to the enemy. The provision for health care was brought forward by Lloyd George's Liberal Government in 1911. Osler was not only a supporter of the Liberal Party, but had spoken once at least at a political meeting, sharing the platform with a local candidate. It would have been quite in character for Osler to have advised the Government on this matter. I have no direct evidence for this, but one curious matter has the Osler stamp. In the legislation for health insurance there was particular emphasis on treatment and prevention of tuberculosis, a favorite of Osler's. This famous legislation, eventually to evolve to become our British National Health Service, was rushed and incomplete because of pressure of other events, and in this may have been the perfect opportunity for the opportunist Osler. In the section on the management of tuberculosis in the new health scheme, there is a provision, unusual for the time, for funding research into tuberculosis. This remarkable little 'bottom slice' was to grow and grow. It was the first government money for any research, and was allowed to grow, eventually becoming the grant for a new Medical Research Council, responsible for the entire British biomedical research effort, then and now. I labor this point to suggest that not only did Osler have a hand in the beginnings of our health service, but if I am right, (and he wrote or inspired or induced Thomas Clifford Allbutt, Regius Professor at Cambridge, who was also an advisor to the government, to write the little section about his favourite disease), then Osler, also had a hand in the foundation of our Medical Research Council.

Important though this was, one other issue soon had Osler back in the thick of medical matters and public debate, in a matter which was much to his heart, and was only brought to a completion shortly before his death. There was great discontent about the hospitals in London, not for the first time nor the last. There were too many hospitals, too many doctors, and the standards, particularly of teaching, could be poor. A great Royal Commission was set up, one of the last of these great Victorian investigations, and Osler was invited to give evidence to it. These commissions, now gone, were a notable part of British life, and allowed serious-minded persons to advise governments on important non-urgent matters. The publication of the Reports was also on a grand scale, since not only the detailed conclusions and proposals were printed, but the verbatim evidence was also published. Osler's experience in Canada and America were vital to the enquiry, and he vigorously championed his view, based on the experience at Hopkins.

Osler gave his evidence in 1911, and prefaced it with his views as given in a lecture to the Northumberland and Durham Medical Society shortly before. The Commission then questioned him, and it is a rare record of Osler speaking extempore. Not quite the only one: he gave similar evidence to the Commission on Vivisection, as Cushing noticed in his biography. Osler's prose is concise and crisp, and not without humor. When asked about the obstacles to his scheme for the London hospitals, he had this exchange with the Chairman, Lord Haldane of Clone. Haldane asks Osler if academic clinical units could be set up.

> Q11.432. Now the next point I come to is the practical possibilities [of the London units].
> How far is it practical?
> *Osler:* I think there is only one difficulty.
> *Haldane:* Money?
> *Osler:* Money.[2]

Osler's proposals were to reduce the number of clinical teaching units in London and join them to the University, thus replacing the master/junior apprentice system prevailing at the time. His innovation was for salaried middle grade doctors, and his scheme for these units, was familiar from his Hopkins days.[3]

Osler's 'University Unit'
—Head/Professor
—Senior Assistants (salaried, full-time)
—House Physician/Surgeon
—Out-patient Clinic Assistants
—Laboratory Assistant/Research

The units were to have about one hundred beds. The additions, the novelties for Britain, were the introduction of the salaried full-time assistants between the existing master and lowly pupil, and the introduction of the laboratory assistants. The crucial debate was about the role of the head of the department—the professor—and we are perhaps surprised that Osler did not propose full-time heads of the units, but instead part-time posts only—mornings only. Osler is associated with the full-time debate, but it is sometimes forgotten that he did not support early proposals for full-time heads of departments. I think this was an entirely pragmatic approach at the time. He often spoke of the 'Utopian idea' that a head of a unit could be found who would be happy taking a salary only. Osler knew that a successful doctor at that time would always be one sought out by rich clients, ready to pay the fees appropriate to their wealth, and Osler was pessimistic that a group of London doctors could be found to give up the chance of private practice and take full-time salaried positions.[4,5] The situation in Germany was returned to time and time again. Carl Harko von Noorden in Vienna seems to have been the most popular specialist of the time, and at the Royal Commission hearing, Osler replied to Haldane,

> Q11.421. *Osler:* When a man gets a reputation such as von Noorden has had in recent years it is very difficult for him to be kept away from people who seek him.
> *Haldane:* You have to reckon with the millionaires?
> *Osler:* Yes. it [full-time work] is quite impossible.[2]

Osler had a private reservation about full-time heads of departments in any case. He thought that after forty that personal innovation was declining, and that the head's role was in general supervision rather than executive action. Indeed, we see that his hope for research lay in the under forties; the hopes for London lay with the salaried assistants. The units were to be in five of the twelve London teaching hospitals then existing.

Medical and Surgical Units
Board of Education proposals
St. Bartholomew's
St. Thomas's
University College
The London Hospital
The Royal Free

The Royal Commission finished its work and published in 1911.[2] But the prospect of war prevented any further implementation of the proposals, and Osler had to await his chance.

World War One

But the War gave Osler a further set of opportunities touching on research and medical progress. The prospect of a war distressed Osler, and was to bring him personal tragedy, but he agreed that the conflict was a necessary one. He had hoped that such barbarism was being eliminated in civilized countries.

But it was a time of opportunity for him; he was ahead of his time and a great supporter of government initiatives. In May 1918, in an unguarded moment at the Royal Society of Medicine, he blurted out,

> [There is] in certain quarters an invincible prejudice against State aid. It is an academic obsession, peculiarly insular and Anglican. . . . There are no grounds whatever for this distrust . . . in the field of infections practically all the first-hand discoveries . . . have been made by men in official harness, such as Griffith Evans, [Patrick] Manson, [Ronald] Ross, [David] Bruce, [William Boog] Leishman and others. The debt of the profession is one-hundred-fold greater to the Local Government Board for its researches in preventive medicine than to all our universities combined.[6]

In a nation at war, practical decisions need to be taken quickly by men of opinion and influence. Osler was in the inner councils of the Establishment. His informal powerful circle included Lord Haldane, Sir George Newman, General Sir Alfred Keogh, and Sir Walter M. Fletcher, secretary of the now-growing Medical Research Council. He memoed and lobbied for schemes which were desirable in peacetime and would succeed in the war, and a remarkable number they were. I list them:

Osler's Wartime Projects
Post-graduate Education

Better Army Medical Records
A History of the War
Better Statistical Returns
Specialist Hospitals
Reform of London Medical Schools
Medical Research Council Expansion

The war offered remarkable opportunities. The collectivism of war places higher priority on the community and public good. The health of the ordinary members of the armed forces is a priority. The doctors in the military are salaried, practising on the basis of need. For the young doctors in World War One the need for post-graduate education was self-evident: large numbers of young men were in the army medical services, and had unfamiliar problems to deal with—infectious diseases, and multiple trauma—unseen in civilian life. The need for education above and beyond the student level was obvious. The presence of many North American units with time available and the challenge of the war gave the necessary environment. Osler organized much informal teaching during the war, and in 1919 set up the first meeting of the Post-graduate Medical Association. Another of Osler's projects was the keeping of good medical records, case studies which followed the military patient through different centers, which although self-evident now, was not then. War offers opportunities for study of disease over prolonged periods in the young, fit, and locatable. Follow-up of disease was uncommon in civilian society then, and here was the chance. Osler lobbied the army, and the now-growing MRC was able to fund this novelty, which civilian medical practice was to follow. He even managed to encourage preparation for a medical history of the war, even when the war was hardly started. He knew that Britain had done little or nothing in the way of compiling a medical history dealing with the earlier campaigns in the Crimea and South Africa. From his antiquarian interests, he was familiar with the remarkable medical history of the Civil War in America, and he urged the War Office to set up a Medical History of the War, and the consulting editors were chosen with Osler himself involved.

Special Hospitals

Osler's unerring instinct for what would work led him to lobby for specialist hospitals. This topic had been a favorite with him earlier at the Royal Commission. In response to a question from Lord Haldane, Osler replied,

> Q11.475. *Osler:* Several of the large Paris hospitals now assign certain wards to certain subjects; to stomach diseases and heart diseases.
> *Haldane:* Your idea would be to have special clinics in each of those departments? It would seem to me at first blush to mean a very great

rearrangement in the distribution of teaching in London.
Osler: Undoubtedly.[2]

The medical profession's instinct was always to resist these subdivisions, but Osler saw opportunities in the war for specialist study of heart research and went for it, encouraging what was known then as the Mount Vernon Heart Hospital.

The War Office however, strongly discouraged any idea of setting apart hospitals for special complaints. It seemed hopeless, but finally Osler, Sir Thomas Clifford Allbutt, Sir James Mackenzie the cardiologist, and Sir Walter Morley Fletcher together bearded Keogh in his den; and 'this did the trick'. In an April 1916 letter to William Sydney Thayer, he wrote,

> We have started a big Army Heart-Hospital [Hampstead]. Allbutt, Mackenzie & I have had the selection of staff & have been put in control as active consultants. . . . [Thomas] Lewis has one [clinic], [Sir John] Parkinson & [Jonathan C.] Meakins (of Montreal) the other, & we hope to be able to get [Frances] Fraser for the 4th.[7]

Hospital Reform

It was only at the end of the war that the earlier schemes for London hospitals resurfaced, and all concerned moved towards implementing the Royal Commission proposals, namely medical and surgical units in selected hospitals; Osler now seventy years old, was unwell and perhaps aware that he had little time left. In a July 1919 letter to Sir George Newman, Osler wrote,

> I had hoped to be able to come up tomorrow, but I am so hoarse that I think it would be safer not to. I have written to [Sir William S.] McCormick [University Grants Committee] urging that the committee approve of the immediate formation of clinical units at Bart's, London, University College & St. Thomas's. The Royal Free people should also be encouraged to proceed at once.[8]

Osler died shortly afterwards in December 1919. Most of his wartime schemes prospered after his death. Postgraduate education flourished, record keeping and follow-up of cases became the norm. The Medical Research Council grew and grew. But his main exploit failedthe establishment of proper medical and surgical units with research interests in London. The London Hospital Units faltered from the first. Some appointments were made, but some directors pulled out immediately. There were muddles about money and control, and supporters like the MRC pulled out. The hospital units at the London teaching hospitals were almost all failures, and eventually dispersed. Only at University College did the desired type of unit emerge under Thomas Lewis. But Lewis was an unusual man, and probably had enough private income to allow himself to be uninterested in medical practice. It was in Scotland and elsewhere that the university departments were to emerge and in London it was at Hammersmith, under Frances Fraser, one of Osler's heart men, that the first viable post-graduate departments and a research hospital arose.

The Aftermath

Osler's skills as negotiator and fixer were missed. Matters became even worse in the 1920s. The MRC turned against support of any medical research by the doctors. One of Osler's circle, Sir Walter Morley Fletcher, now Secretary of the MRC, brought in a strict policy of giving funds entirely to support basic science, arguing that from that source only came future medical advances. The failure of the London units was used to justify this policy. This rift between the scientists and clinicians widened and became public. Lords Moynihan and Dawson, eminent clinicians, openly attacked the MRC in 1933, and the MRC retaliated in trying to thwart clinical research fund-raising, notably by the cancer charities.

The archives of the time show may bitter exchanges between the doctors and the scientists and MRC, in the struggle for the scarce resources. Fletcher attempted to prevent the setting up of the British Empire Cancer Campaign. He wrote that "research was too difficult for doctors,"

> a committee of eminent clinicians will be perfectly useless . . . if these men really want to help they ought to preach in season and out of season to their rich clients and to the general public the essential importance of maintained [basic research] work along the line and not only in particular frontal attacks . . .

No one in the 1920s had emerged with Osler's skills and diplomacy.

Going back to the original question of Osler's attitude to medical research, there is no doubt that he actively supported medical research and development, and sought to set up mechanisms whereby the best teachers and researchers were encouraged and given their opportunity in their prime to use their talents. I think he considered that research was crucial, but had its limits. In his address 'The Leaven of Science', he pointed out that science could achieve much, but had little impact on the eternal role of the doctor as a personal advisor. Nor, he thought, did science have much influence on the higher or lower achievements of the human race. By this he meant that in the matter of sense and sensibility and the arts, scientific advance changed little. He had a second reservation about the worship of scientific progress, since it had not made much impact on the worse of human emotions, and did not in particular seem to soften the aggression of nations. Scientists in Germany had spoken out openly in favor of a war, and they made the ghastly chemical weapons used. Some among the victors suggested that the successful German scientific effort, including their dominance in reductionist medicine, had helped create an amoral society which was doomed, and had been rightly defeated in war.

In summary, Osler had high aims for the medical profession and indeed for mankind. In his verdict on scientific medicine, Osler used a powerful analogy from the bakery. Science within medicine was but a leaven for the maturation of the practice of medicine, an unpalatable and even unpleasant ingredient when taken on its own without the bread. Science was a useful addition, but not the dominant aim for the profession in its ancient and essential role—that of a comforter, healer and friend.

References

1. Cushing, Harvey. *The Life of Sir William Osler.* 2 Vols, Oxford, Clarendon Press, 1925, Vol. 1, p. 331.
2. *Royal Commission on University Education in London.* Appendix to the Third Report, Minutes of Evidence, Cd 1911.
3. Graham, George. The formation of the medical and surgical professorial units in the London teaching hospitals. *Annals of Science* 26: 1-22, 1970.
4. Osler, William. London University Reform, *Quarterly Review* 219: 204-230, 1913.
5. Fleming, Donald. The full-time controversy. *J Med Educ* 30: 398-406, 1955.
6. Op. cit. #1, Cushing, Vol. 2, pp. 605-606.
7. Ibid., Vol. 2, p. 523.
8. Ibid., Vol. 2, p. 664

A Body of Knowledge: Knowledge of the Body*

Sherwin B. Nuland

Sherwin B. Nuland is Clinical Professor of Surgery Emeritus, at the Yale University School of Medicine, where he has been studying and working since starting medical school in 1951. A New York native and a product of city schools, he became interested in history at Public School 33 in the Bronx. He maintained that interest during a thirty-year career in surgery, during which he not only wrote numerous research and clinical papers, but gradually taught himself to be a medical historian. In addition to numerous articles, his books include: *Doctors: The Biography of Medicine* (1989).

In 1994, Dr. Nuland published *How We Die,* a study of the modern way of death, which astonished him by becoming what glib publicists called "a runaway best seller". This monograph has been translated into some fifteen languages, and more than half a million copies have been sold in countries throughout the world. This volume won that year's National Book Award, and was a finalist for the 1995 Pulitzer Prize and Book Critics' Circle Award. More recently he has written *The Wisdom of the Body* (1997), and *How We Live* (1998).

Dr. Nuland has written for the *New Yorker, Discover, The New Republic, Time, The New York Review of Books,* and other periodicals for the general reader.

*Delivered 10 May 1995 at the Twenty-fifth Annual Meeting of the American Osler Society, Pittsburgh, Pennsylvania

Perhaps it is a function of increasing age, but I find myself thinking often these days about the human spirit. Are we indeed greater than the sum of our parts, and is there a quality residing within *Homo sapiens* that distinguishes us, beyond strictly evolutionary characteristics, from all other animals? I mean this in the biological, and not in the theological, sense.

Until recently, I had forgotten that almost ten years ago I had written the following, in the book called *Doctors: The Biography of Medicine*,

> I am convinced that there is a biologically determined characteristic that is the human spirit—that there is a gene or genes for it just as surely as there is a gene or genes for the color of our eyes or the length of our fingers. I have no idea whether it was put in place by the power that some call God or the power that some call chance, but it is reproduced within us with the same predictability as the rising and setting sun. It is not our intellect or even our physical structure that is the criterion of our humanness; man is the most fulfilled animal on this planet because there resides in us the motivating and civilizing force of the human spirit. It gives us the ability to think courageous thoughts, do courageous deeds, and give courageous sustenance to our fellows. I predict that it will one day be the subject of scientific research and validating experiment. . . . I don't believe for a minute that minds capable of solving the mysteries of DNA will not, in some distant future, elucidate what are now seen as the miraculous mysteries of human nature. There are, as Goethe tells us, no miracles; there are only those mysteries of nature, and they wait to be solved.

As late as the middle of the ninteenth century, many authorities, and virtually all plain people too, believed that living things were possessed of an unknowable form of energy that made them vastly different from structures not endowed with life. Because this hypothetical energy was commonly called "the vital force", the scientists and other learned people who trusted in its existence were known as "vitalists." The concept of vitalism stood independent of religious conviction—there was nothing about it that necessarily required a supernatural or theological explanation. Although some vitalists, starting as far back as Aristotle in the fourth century BC, identified the life force in humans with the psyche, many others thought that it had no connection to mind or soul. Obviously, though, there were those of a less scientific bent who embraced vitalism because of their certainty that the unknown and unknowable factor was God-given.

Many of the secular vitalists were persuaded that the origin of the life force was not explainable by the usual principles of physics or chemistry, but some few of the staunchest proponents of the theory maintained, on the other hand, that it would eventually be shown to be regulated by as yet undiscovered natural laws. They reasoned that if this proved to be the case, it might then become possible to carry out laboratory studies of this unique form of energy.

The belief in vitalism, at least among scientists, had lost favor by the latter half of the ninteenth century as biochemical and physiological elucidations of the characteristics of living things increasingly emerged from the burgeoning numbers of research laboratories making their appearance in Europe, and to a lesser extent in North America. The so-called "mechanists," those who sought physicochemical explanations of life processes, had won the battle and convinced all but a few diehards of their correctness.

And yet, the general notion of vitalism, attenuated although it may be, lives on in the minds of any and all who refuse to believe that there is not more to the phenomenon of life than a series of chemical reactions.

Ranged against the principle of vitalism is an array of evidence so overwhelming that twentieth-century scientists have never questioned it. To them, the physicochemical or "mechanistic" view of life has become axiomatic. Even stubborn latter-day vitalists cannot question that at the very least, the mechanistic bases of life become even more evident with each passing decade.

The characteristics shared by all living things can be listed:

Respiration
Circulation
Responsiveness, or Adaptability
Assimilation
Absorption
Digestion
Excretion
Movement
Growth
Reproduction

This list may serve as a perfectly adequate accounting of all the biological functions that characterize living things, but it should not be mistaken for an attempt to define such an abstruse and immensely complex word as *Life.* Life is a concept, a philosophy, an abstraction, a point of view—and also a chimera and a thousand tangibles and intangibles, substantialities and imponderables, appearing quite different from every one of the many angles and along every one of the many axes from which it may be approached.

Even the most detailed mechanistic descriptions of our nuts-and-bolts physicochemistry are missing something, and that something is immense. More than one scientist has expressed frustration with how little is even now known about the *organization* of our biological faculties, functioning with such an integrated degree of coordination that we are capable of what would seem to be mental and physical miracles, not to say spiritual ones, which would appear to transcend the mere interaction of molecules.

Otto Loewi was such a scientist. Loewi was the physiologist who first demonstrated that impulses pass through the gap between nerve cells by means of chemical substances, rather than via an electrical wave as had been previously supposed. There could not have been a more mechanistic laboratory-produced explanation of a phenomenon that for millennia had been presumed a miracle of inscrutable mystery.

But even in the face of his discoveries, something in Loewi refused to give up his fascination with that mystery. He never lost his sparkling ability to indulge in it, and allowed himself to wonder what else there might be. As a scientist he devoted his life to proving that the totality was no more than the sum of its physicochemical parts, but there were playful elves in his soul, and once in a while he would smilingly say the kind of thing reported by his nephew: "The beauty of the Budapest String Quartet can never be explained by a little acetylcholine in the nerves and muscles." After his death in 1961 at the age of 89, Loewi was quoted by his nephew as having believed that "the life sciences contain spiritual values which can never be explained by the materialistic attitude of present-day science."

Not all of science, of course, is materialistic—and very few scientists are cynical about the sources of life. Not infrequently, some of the self-same researchers whose career-long work it is to seek out materialistic or mechanistic answers, are precisely those most urgently questing after the secret sources of the mysteries; the very wonderment that sustains the ceaseless curiosity of so many researchers is precisely their wonderment at the marvels of nature. Otto Loewi has never been alone in his awe. To search for a biochemical or physical basis for those marvels is not to lessen that awe. In some ways the awe is greater in fact, when it can be shown that no magic is needed to elucidate one or another of nature's closet-secrets. That enormously complex biological interactions are so flawlessly coordinated as to result in such obvious manifestations as human thought is as exciting to me—actually more exciting—than such phenomena were when I was a small boy and thought them divinely driven.

What I find most exhilarating is not even the freedom from invoking magic that modern science provides. As paradoxical as it may at first sound coming out of the mouth of a skeptic like me, the ultimate exhilaration derives from my conviction that the whole *is* greater than the sum of its parts.

In my view, humankind has adapted to the surroundings in which it finds itself in ways far greater than the mere evolutionary or physicochemical events might have decreed. The physicochemical and genetic may have provided us the basic ability to *integrate* our mental and somatic functioning, and they may also have given us the inborn ability to adapt, but the very way in which we have made use of that adaptability is the real secret of how our species has transcended the limitations that even our extraordinary molecular function impose on us.

The anatomy of intricate circuitry in our brains and the balance of hormonal controls in our physiology can take us only so far. Millennium by millennium, *Homo sapiens* has, I believe, built up patterns of anticipatory thought and reflection, and evolved a culture that could not have been predicted relying only on knowledge of our anatomy and physiology. It is necessary to take other factors into account.

To us must go the credit for using our inborn neurological connections and cerebral centers to bring about the real creation—the creation of humanity from *Homo*. By the way, we have gradually brought ourselves to *utilize* the nature-given complex of molecules and wires we piecemeal over eons, and discovered the pathways and linkages within us to develop the qualities of abstract thinking that are the hallmark of our species.

We have sent exploring couriers in the form of electrical impulses, up and down the cerebral highways and into remote junctions, paths, and way-stations. They have returned after finding linkages and routes that we then employed to provide us with memory, foresight, and reflection. With memory, foresight, and reflection we were able to build a logical pattern of evaluating the evidence of our senses and employing it in decision-making. That power might not necessarily have arisen, although the strictly physical equipment for it was in place. By a process of chance, by trial and error, by firing and misfiring among the ten billion brain cells and their thousand times that many connections to each other (amounting to some ten trillion in all), we have made unanticipated albeit not consciously recognized discoveries and thereby adapted to what nature originally gave us with the intention only of helping us to survive and reproduce.

In coming upon and utilizing a myriad of local electrical circuits organized into interconnecting regions and systems in our brains, and by turning our hormonal capabilities to uses beyond the basic needs of passing on the DNA, we have created humanity and all that humanity represents. By this I mean not only the concept of social relationships and community, but what is more basic—hope, faith, altruism, obligation, charity, morality and even those aspects of love that are selfless and non-procreative. We have gone so far as to create enriching qualities that are totally useless for survival, most particularly our esthetic sensibility, manifest in our appreciation of beauty and our need for order. Certainly the *capacities* for developing those characteristics which we recognize as uniquely human came originally with the molecular equipment assigned to us by natural selection, but it is through *Homo sapiens'* gradual explorations and discoveries that the capacity became reality. This then is the ultimate process by which the human spirit has come into being. It is in the way we have made use of our innate physiology and anatomy that we ourselves, the members of our own species, are the real creators.

I refer here to actual organic events, to messages that move along nerve fibres and cells that respond to the stimuli thus induced. It should not be thought that I am presenting a rehash of psychological theory. In my view, contemporary psychology is in itself a form of vitalism, postulating psychic energy of an immeasurable nature and a mind that functions in some ways independently of the demonstrable physiology of the brain. On the other hand, though, I do not so much dismiss the notion of certain bulwarks of psychoanalytic thought, as I seek to explicate them on an organic basis.

In his masterly *Civilization and Its Discontents,* Sigmund Freud postulates that in addition to the personal superego, humankind has developed what might be called a cultural superego. Personal superego "commands and prohibits" in the manner of an internalized father like authority figure (equated with conscience); cultural superego forces the individual into behavior patterns that conform to the values of the surrounding society. In an expanded sense, the cultural superego forces the society itself to act much like an individual, overseen by generally accepted ethical precepts. As Freud puts it, "That which began in relation to the father ends in relation to the community!" Clearly, the demands of the superego and cultural superego largely coincide, with the difference that the superego is subconscious. The essential message here is that on every level, from the subconscious to the communal, we absorb the rules laid down by the authority structure into whose realms we enter.

I do not believe that any of this is a "psychological" process, if by psychological is meant the mind as distinct from the brain. I suspect that the elemental brain of *Homo sapiens* was, and is, the repository of vast quantities of excess circuitry and cellular structure, just as the rest of the body has vast quantities of excess hormonal and other capacity. Nature everywhere provides its creatures with plenty of reserves of cells, tissues, and even organs—we do not really need two kidneys, or such a perfectly huge liver, among other examples. Over tens of thousands of years, we have adapted to the dangers and rewards associated with the basic genetically determined instincts we share with all life, namely self-preservation and reproduction. In order to adapt to the constantly changing circumstances of everyday existence, every organism has used some of its excess capacity, but the reserve capacity, at least the cerebral reserve capacity, of humans is immensely greater than that of any other creatures. Thanks to our extraordinary neocortex, our ability to adapt in the intellectual and emotional sense is capacious, and almost certainly even now underutilized. Adapting and responding to sensory input from the body and its surroundings, delivered over incoming fibres and via chemical messengers, the human brain has engaged itself in the instinctual battle between *Eros* and *Thanatos*—the forces of love (and therefore life) against the forces of the death instinct. Because the two are irreconcilable, the central nervous system of man had, since the time it originally came into existence with the birth of the first *Homo sapiens*, to conjure with itself—to try various combinations of circuitry and chemistry, and to turn to its excess reserve capacity in exploratory ways—until it became what it is today, a vast machine works of intellect, spirituality, and even neurosis.

The process is hit or miss: chance firings, misfirings, electrical journeys made, electrical journeys aborted or rerouted anywhere along the way, and gradually the establishment of message routes that seem most suitable to the needs of the therefore ever more intellectually capable human being. As these newly discovered pathways are more frequently traveled, the passage of messages along them becomes easier and easier until it is at last virtually automatic, while the resulting thought and behavioral patterns become the accepted characteristics of the person. The ever enlarging set of responses is so internalized after a while that offspring effortlessly learn it from their parents and surroundings during the long period of early human childhood.

Perhaps the greatest feat of this humanizing process is the recognition of beauty, both the beauty we find around us and the beauty we can create. Beauty in and of itself is of no consequence to the DNA's survival needs, and that alone makes its recognition one of the supreme accomplishments of the human mind, beauty of image, of sound, of thought—give us the sense of enrichment, even of spirituality, that goes well beyond our constant seeking of mere survival and pleasure. The human spirit and its perpetual search for beauty are the defining characteristics of our humanity.

In my book *How We Die* (1994), I discussed the necessity that the life of each of us must come to an end. Were it not for our individual deaths, I opined, civilization would stagnate, life could not renew itself with enthusiastic vigor in each generation, and the world, as Tennyson put it, "would grow moldy, would only breed the past again." Nevertheless, that does not answer the question of why it is biologically necessary that living things must die. If all our inborn biological drives serve in one way or another the twin purposes of self-preservation and reproduction, where does death fit in? On what mechanistic or physiologic basis do psychoanalytic theorists dare to propose the existence not only of the life-enhancing quality of *Eros*, but also of *Thanatos*? The entire principle of natural selection presupposes that all forms of life are imperfect, and that the causes of their deaths are the result, either directly or indirectly, of those imperfections. But that in itself does not necessitate an actual instinct that drives us toward dying in the way in which the more overt instinicts of *Eros* drive us toward living.

It is precisely in the matter of death that our notions of instinct and even molecular biology still fail us. Although there is some preliminary evidence of cells being destroyed by what is currently being called a "death gene", much must still be done before its workings are elucidated. Almost paradoxically, the "death gene" appears to be an agency of the very forces that preserve life. Killing groups of cells when they have outlived their usefulness serves the purpose of progressive development of the entire organism, as well as keeping it alive.

I am intrigued by a statement made earlier in this century by the eminent medical historian and physician, Logan Clendening. In his hugely popular 1927 book, *The Human Body,* Clendening wrote, "strictly speaking, death is not a biological necessity. There is no inherent reason any cell should ever die." Not at all a man of religious faith, Clendening followed this with, "As I think it over, death seems to me one of the few evidences in nature of the operation of a creative intelligence: of an intelligence exhibiting qualities which I recognize as mind stuff. To have blundered on the form of energy called life showed a sort of malignant power. After having blundered on life, to have conceived of death was a real stroke of a genius."

As a free-thinker, Clendening seems to have meant this ironically, if not actually with a tinge of sarcasm. He was referring to the "genius" of mindless nature, creating the marvel of life simply by the random juxtaposition of atoms, molecules, and explosive energy at a coincidence of timing, and then going on to develop mechanisms to insure the survival and propagation of those marvels—even if it requires their individual destruction in each generation. In Clendening's scheme and in mine, the genius of having conceived it lies in the fact that death is the guarantor of the perpetuation of life.

What life has become for our species is, I believe, the result of the way we have adapted to our environment by discovering ways to utilize the surplus potentiality of our neural and endocrine selves. The reason natural selection provides a surplus is self-evident. An injured creature is more likely to survive and reproduce if it has a surplus to fall back on. Perhaps the very bilaterality of animals is the result of such a selectivity, providing paired organs and even considerable extras in such single structures as liver, spleen, and intestines—and of course brain. It is to adaptive use of the considerable extras in the endocrine and central nervous systems, I believe, that we owe our discovery of the mechanisms whereby we created the human spirit.

Seen this way, the human spirit is a generated product of our innate biology. Born with the biologic extras and resources to create, we have done just that. Whether the process by which it has been created is one of millennia-long adaptation, or is primarily a gene-driven process, as I once thought—the endpoint of all is that it exists as a product of our molecules. Nothing more need be sought. There is no need to invoke either a higher power or magic. We need only invoke what is in our human cells, the highest power and the greatest magic that has ever awed a wonder-struck observer of its magnificence.

There is no end to the series of adaptations along whose continuum we now find ourselves. Barring world or species-destroying catastrophe, the cerebral circuits and the neuroendocrine interactions will never stop discovering new ways to deal with the stimuli presented to them, and will accordingly never stop enhancing our capacity to solve the puzzles inherent in the physical and mental challenges that constantly surround us.

It might be pointed out, and properly so, that all of this presupposes a state of constant improvement, and therefore presents Pollyanna's view of the human mind and its potentialities. But I do not restrict myself to the *sublime* qualities developed within our species. In my definition of the human spirit is included those other characteristics of which we are far less proud, the base qualities in all that is subsumed under the rubric of humanness. If there is an antonym for everything we customarily associate with *spiritual,* it must surely be *mean-spirited.* The same adaptive use of circuitry and molecular interactions that allows humankind to perform the mental gymnastics leading to our firtest accomplishments is also in thrall to our baser instincts.

After all, the biological imperative of our existence is survival. Of what survival value is the human spirit? Why have we endlessly prowled the thousands of miles of our cerebral connections in search of every aspect of it? The answer is that the human spirit enhances and enriches life. The very fact that life can be pleasurable makes us more likely to seek out atmospheres and behaviors that tend to increase the probability that it will not end. But like all adaptations, some arc *mal*adaptive. The maladaptations, the conflict between the instinctual forces of *Eros* and *Thanatos*, and the interplay of such factors with the stresses of everyday life—these are the stuff of antisocial behavior and neurosis. They will always exist, and they too are part of what makes us human.

Again and again, the notion of *instincts* has appeared in this discussion. A word variously interpreted by the philosopher, the psychologic theorist, and the laboratory scientist, there would seem to be a general agreement on a basic formulation provided by the lexicographer. My Webster puts it this way: **Instinct:** an inborn tendency to behave in a way characteristic of a species; natural unacquired mode of response to stimuli; as, suckling is an *instinct* in mammals.

The word is derived from the Latin compound verb *instinguere,* to urge onward or impel *(instigate* obviously has the same origin), constructed from the prefix *in* (on) and *stinguere* (goad, or prick). The involuntary aspect of the word's implications is clear, especially when *stinguere* is traced to its Indo-European root, which is *steig,* meaning prick, or pointed, or sharp. In the mid-sixteenth century, instinct acquired its current usage as "an innate impulse" or an inborn tendency specific to a particular species.

Seeking an up-to-the minute scientific or perhaps mechanistic interpretation of what is meant by instinct, we might turn to the recent brilliant *tour-de-force* of the neurobiologist Antonio Damasio, *Descartes' Error,* in which he points out early in a chapter titled *Biological Regulation and Survival* that "the brain has innate neural circuits whose activity patterns, assisted by biochemical processes in the body proper, reliably control reflexes, drives and instincts, and thus ensure that respiration and feeding are implemented as needed. . . . On another front, to avoid destruction by predators or adverse environmental conditions, there are neural circuits for drives and instincts that cause, for example, fight or flight behaviors. Still others control drives and instincts that help ensure the continuation of the individual's genes. . . . In general, drives and instincts operate either by generating a particular behavior directly or by inducing [e.g. by means of hormones] physiological states that lead individuals to behave in a particular way, mindlessly or not."

In other words, although we may or may not be aware that they are functioning ("mindlessly or not"), instinctual behaviors are inborn and driven—in a more basic sense the result of goading and pricking. Whether we consciously want to or not, our innate drives goad and prick us toward staying alive and reproducing ourselves.

Where in this formulation is the prized quality we call reason, and what is its source? Like other of our self-created qualities, reason gently leavens those patterns of instinctual behavior that are inimical to the highest motivations and yearnings of the human spirit. Unlike that other self-creation, superego or conscience, it is not harsh or punishing. Reason, in fact, often mediates between drives and conscience, to lessen the cruelty that might otherwise be inflicted by an overly strict and destructive superego. As the poet George Herbert put it in 1640, "Reason lies between the spur and the bridle."

Although reason is often required to fight the worst moral qualities of instinct, and to mitigate the sternest judgment of conscience, the three are best employed in an alliance under reason's leadership. Bertrand Russell has written that his notion of morality is one in which "instinct should be trained rather than thwarted." Reason is the trainer.

But even here our creations are imperfect. The very power of reason that we employ to understand and sweeten our lives, we employ also in the pursuit of objectives more in keeping with the demands of our less-than-ideally trained instincts. We confuse reason with rationalization, and betray our highest spiritual values. In *Uncle Vanya,* Anton Chekhov has Constantin say, "Man has been endowed with reason, with the power to create, so that he can add to what he's been given. But up to now he hasn't been a creator, only a destroyer. Forests keep disappearing, rivers dry up, wild life's become extinct, the climate's ruined and the land grows poorer and uglier every day."

I would modify Chekhov's first sentence, to say that man has discovered the neurological pathways and learned to use the hormonal interactions which he has then employed in the creation of reason. By using reason, both consciously and subconsciously he has made even more neural and biochemical discoveries with which he is constantly creating new aspects of humanness and expanding the horizons of his spirit. Unfortunately, he has not seldom used his capacity of self-creation to allow himself to accede to drives of destructiveness, either in his inner or communal life. In this way have neuroses been created and sources of buoyant life suppressed. Such considerations bring some hesitation to our acceptance of the psalmist's encomium that we are "a little lower than the angels, and crowned with glory and honor."

It is my spiritual self that makes me human. It enables me to reason, to sublimate my instinctual drives, to be of use to society, and to love in the way that only a member of my species can love; it enables me to do harm, to scheme against the interests of others, and to so misinterpret the subconsciously recalled traumas of my childhood that I become depressed, anxious, or a danger to society. The human spirit can be the high road to the fulfillment of my greatest hopes; it can be the grim pathway to my self-destruction.

Other People's Bodies: Human Experimentation on the Fiftieth Anniversary of the Nuremberg Code*

David J. Rothman

David J. Rothman is Bernard Schoenberg Professor of Social Medicine and Director of the Center for the Study of Society and Medicine at the Columbia College of Physicians and Surgeons, and Professor of History at Columbia University.

Educated in social history at Harvard University, he has explored American practices toward the deviant and dependent. His study of the origins of mental hospitals, prisons, and almshouses, *The Discovery of the Asylum* (1971), was co-winner of the Albert J. Beveridge Prize of the American History Association. He continued tracing these events in *Conscience and Convenience: The Asylum and Its Alternatives in Progressive America* (1980). Together with Sheila M. Rothman, he published *The Willowbrook Wars'* (1984), *Children's Hospitals in the Progressive Era* (1987), and *Redesigning the Self: The Promise and Perils of Genetic Enhancement* (2002). Other works include *Strangers at the Bedside; A History of How Law and Bioethics Transformed Medical Decision-making* (1991), *The Oxford History of the Prison* (1996, co-edited with Norval Morris), and *Beginnings Count: The Technological Imperative in American Health Care* (1997).

In 1983, he joined the Columbia Medical School faculty. His recent work has addressed issues in the history of human experimentation, the history of drug regulation and clinical trials with a particular focus on AIDS, and the rationing of scarce medical resources. Dr. Rothman is co-director of the Columbia-Montefiore Certificate Program in Bioethics and the Medical Humanities, he is a member of the Board of Trustees of the Open Society Institute, and

*Delivered 25 April 1996, at the Twenty-sixth Annual Meeting of the American Osler Society, San Francisco, California

a member of the Board of Advisors of the Project on Death in America of that Institute.

He is recipient of the Albert J. Beveridge prize of the American Historical Association (1971). In 1987, he received an honorary Doctor of Law Degree from the John Jay School of Criminal Justice.

In the fifty years since the issuance of the Nuremberg Code, the ethics of human experimentation has assumed such centrality in social thought and public policy that it requires an act of imagination to recall just how novel this event was. Nuremberg represented the first attempt to set forth and enforce an explicit set of principles, literally a code, in the conduct of human experimentation. Whatever weaknesses commentators would later identify, and whatever refinements marked the content of successor codes, Nuremberg was the pioneer effort to implement standards that clinical investigators were required to observe.[1]

Its originality as a code notwithstanding, Nuremberg was certainly not the earliest effort to analyze the ethics of human experimentation. Already in the thirteenth century, the English philosopher Roger Bacon had explained that progress in medicine would never come as quickly as in the natural sciences because scientists could "multiply their experiments till they get rid of deficiency and errors." The physician, on the other hand, was unable to do this "because of the nobility of the material in which he works."[2] Over the years, many individuals proposed appropriate standards for investigators to follow and decried particular abuses in practice. But until Nuremberg, there was practically no professional or public governance of human experimentation.

Thus, to appreciate the degree to which Nuremberg built on past precedents and the degree to which it represented a novel departure, it is necessary to examine the state of clinical research and ethics before 1947. First, in terms of principles, what obligations did investigator owe the subject? What information was to be shared? What degree of consent, if any, was necessary? Second, in terms of practice, were the principles respected by investigators? Did they live up to the standards? Finally, to the extent that practice diverged from principle, what efforts were made at enforcing standards? Were penalties levied on errant researchers, either by legally constituted bodies or professional organizations?

All of these questions are of obvious relevance to the history of medicine. But no less important, particularly as we observe this fiftieth anniversary, they are essential to framing the contribution of the Nuremberg Code itself.[3] At the trial of the Nazi doctors, defense attorneys claimed that before World War II the ethics of human experimentation were undeveloped, both in the United States and Germany. Principles of voluntariness and of consent, they argued, were poorly understood and usually ignored. American physicians, no less than German ones, paid no heed to consent and frequently carried out experiments on ignorant and unwilling subjects. These points certainly establish Nuremberg's novelty, but at the price of finding a fatal flaw in the prosecution of the Nazi doctors. Nuremberg becomes an exercise in *ex post facto* punishment, setting new standards and then imposing them on the defendants. To be sure, the conviction and punishment of the offenders could easily be justified by ruling that their acts were so horrendous that they constituted a crime against humanity. They had committed war crimes, including the murder of innocent civilians; indeed, the Nuremberg court offered this very judgment: "The record clearly shows the commission of war crimes and crimes against humanity." But instead of stopping there it continued on to address the issue of "Permissible Medical Experiments." Ultimately, it condemned the Nazi doctors for unethical research; they were guilty as physicians, not as civilians, of "violating moral, ethical and legal concepts," not in a more straightforward sense, of murder. Precisely why the court eschewed war crimes and addressed human experimentation as such has never been satisfactorily explained. But whatever the reason, the court's posture brought unprecedented attention to the ethics of human experimentation.

Ethical Principles in Human Experimentation Before Nuremberg

The modern history of the ethics of human experimentation begins with Claude Bernard's 1865 book, *An Introduction to the Study of Experimental Medicine.* No one more cogently than Bernard delineated the potential contribution that clinical research could make to medicine. So vital was it that Bernard regarded experimentation as the third pillar of medical knowledge. As he traced it, physicians first based their treatments upon findings made through their senses, that is, what they saw and heard through direct and intimate encounters with the patient. They felt the pulse, noted the color of the face, examined the urine, and listened to the chest, initially by putting their ear to it, later by using a stethoscope. Physicians, Bernard continued, learned to do more than rely upon their senses. They also "observed," by which he meant that they grouped facts together and formulated hypotheses; they made predictions about treatment outcomes and then studied whether they proved right. In this way, observation was essential to determining which interventions were effective. From Bernard's perspective, however, this exercise was essentially passive. The physician stood back and collected data, wisely and shrewdly, but from a distance.

It was the third form of knowledge that Bernard celebrated, what might be called "active observation." To clarify its meaning and implications, Bernard invoked the French naturalist, Georges Cuvier: "The observer listens to nature; the experimenter questions [nature] and forces her to unveil herself." In his own terms,

> Experimenters must be able to touch the body on which they act, whether by destroying it or by altering it, so as to learn the part which it plays in the phenomena of nature. . . . It is on this very possibility of acting, or not acting, on a body that the distinction will exclusively rest between sciences called sciences of observation and sciences called experimental.

The very language with which Bernard describes experimentation establishes its potency, not only in terms of its ability to create knowledge but to generate ethical problems as well. Bernard's experimenter "touches" parts of the body, not gently, but to destroy it or alter it so as to learn more about its biological function. In this way, the investigator forces nature to "unveil herself," and in the process, he himself becomes an aggressor, indeed, something of a molester as he strips nature of her secrets.[4]

Had Bernard stopped his analysis of clinical research there, the development of human experimentation in the nineteenth century would appear as an exercise in the ruthless accumulation of knowledge, one that was deaf to the decencies of humanity or principles of ethics. But Bernard went on, and after exploring the epistemology and methods of clinical research, he declared in passages now famous,

> Experiments, then, may be performed on man, but within what limits? It is our duty and our right to perform an experiment on man whenever it can save his life, cure him or gain him some benefit. The principle of medical and surgical morality, therefore, consists in never performing on man an experiment which might be harmful to him to any extent, even though the result might be highly advantageous to science, i.e., to the health of others.

Bernard provides a frank and full recognition of the power of human experimentation to do good and to do harm. And with this double-edged potential in mind, he insists that research must always be in the best interests of the subject. If an experiment has the potential to cure, it may be carried out. But if it has no therapeutic potential and may injure the subject, it must not be conducted, regardless of how important the findings might be for others.

Obviously, Bernard's maxims are not fully in accord with contemporary principles, particularly given the scant attention he paid to the idea and meaning of consent. But others among his contemporaries not only echoed his insightful judgments but on occasion went beyond them, incorporating principles of consent into their own frameworks.

This was certainly true of the great clinician, William Osler. Properly credited with bringing scientific methods into medical education and clinical practice,

Osler, as would be expected, was fully appreciative of the vital role of human experimentation. In 1907, he addressed "The Evolution of the Idea of Experiment in Medicine," sounding very much like Claude Bernard, and when it came to consent, superseding him.[5]

Like Bernard, Osler emphasized both the enormous capacity of clinical medicine to generate new knowledge and its highly invasive characteristics. In his formulation, "Man can interrogate as well as observe nature," and through this process, lighten many of "the burdens of humanity." Even more consistently than Bernard, Osler believed that experimentation was part and parcel of the conduct of clinical practice. "Every dose of medicine given is an experiment as it is impossible in every instance to predict what the result may be. "Even so, he, too, insisted on setting limits on human experimentation. First, experiments on man must never be carried out before they had been tried on animals. Second, and here he departed from Bernard, Osler not only ruled out non-therapeutic research but required investigators to obtain the consent of the subject,

> For man absolute safety and full consent are the conditions which make such tests allowable. We have no right to use patients entrusted to our care for the purpose of experimentation unless direct benefit to the individual is likely to follow. Once this limit is transgressed, the sacred cord which binds physician and patient snaps instantly.

In effect, Osler enunciated the principles of consent well in advance of this proposition in the Nuremberg Code.

The viewpoints expressed by Bernard and Osler were shared widely. In 1886, a less prominent Boston physician, Charles Francis Withington, published an essay entitled, *The Relation of Hospitals to Medical Education.*[6] The position he advocated was regarded as so important that his contribution won the prestigious Boylston Prize from Harvard University. Withington posed the ethical question in terms of the "possible conflict between the interests of medical science and those of the individual patient, and the latter's indefeasible rights." He was not at all confident that investigators satisfactorily resolved the conflict, and in truth, he himself had some trouble drawing boundaries between the needs of science and the "rights" (his term) of patients. But in the end, he came down staunchly on the side of rights, to the point of suggesting a remedy of a patient "Bill of Rights" which would not be adopted for another ninety years,

> In the older countries of Europe especially, where the life and happiness of the so-called lower classes are perhaps held more cheaply than with us, enthusiastic devotees of science are very apt to encroach upon the rights of the individual patient in a manner which cannot be justified. In this country, we are less likely to fall into this error than those living

> under monarchical institutions, but even with us it may be well to draw up, as it were, a Bill of Rights which shall secure patients against any injustice from the votaries of science.

Withington insisted that patients had "a right to immunity from experiments merely *as such,* and outside the therapeutic application. This right is one that is especially liable to violation by enthusiastic investigators." Researchers who wished to try a new drug had to rely upon volunteers. In his view, "They had no right to make any man the unwilling victim of such an experiment." Withington was also alert to the possibilities of nontherapeutic experiments on terminally ill patients. An investigator, he insisted, "has no right to take advantage of the patient's extremity to recommend a procedure which can have no other advantage than to enhance the operator's reputation for boldness." He then concluded with a sentence that encapsulated the core principals of medical ethics: "The occupants of hospital wards are something more than merely so much clinical material during their lives and so much pathological material after their death."[6]

Although other texts reiterating these same principles could be easily marshalled, these three make apparent that the ethical dimensions of clinical research were recognized by physicians who advanced the development of modern medicine.[7] Such a conclusion ought not be surprising, for the bedrock principle on which they rested their analyses was as old as medical ethics itself: do no harm, neither to the patient nor to the subject. Experimentation was bound by the ethics of the doctor-patient relationship, which, as we shall see, was a useful starting point, although not an altogether adequate model upon which to base the regulation of human experimentation.

All these writings drew a sharp distinction between therapeutic and nontherapeutic research, and were far more concerned with the latter than the former. They had little difficulty in condemning nontherapeutic research, especially when it placed the subject-patient at risk. But what was almost completely absent from the analysis was a discussion of the ethical principles that should govern experiments with a therapeutic potential. What was the physician obliged to tell the patient about an experiment that might benefit him? Was consent required? Who was to make the calculus of risk of harm versus benefit of cure? By ignoring this set of issues and focusing so exclusively on nontherapeutic research, these commentators make the intent and motive of the physician-researcher the critical determinant. Were he seeking new knowledge and not attempting to benefit the patient, then he was obligated to share information with the subject and obtain consent. But were his intentions to cure or to treat, then apparently he did not have to divulge the facts or obtain the patient's acquiescence to the procedure. Thus, the position adopted (which would remain intact for many decades) was consistent with the tradition in medical ethics of trusting to the integrity of the physician, not requiring formal collegial oversight or consultation or the patient's agreement. So long as the researcher's self-styled purpose was to benefit the patient, he enjoyed an ample discretion unfettered by colleagues or patients. In brief, the mindset of the physician, not the autonomy of the subject, drove the ethical analysis.

The Practice of Human Expermination Before Nuremberg

The uniformity that marked the discussions of the ethical principles in research disappears when one examines the actual practices of investigators, and the reactions to them by the medical profession and the public. Here one finds countless examples of research conduct that blatantly violates the prevailing ethical norms. In a similar vein, one finds some observers outraged by the transgressions and others far more complaisant. The one generalization that can be offered is that no matter how grievous the ethical misconduct in research, professional disciplinary action or some collective expression of censure or disapproval almost never occurred. With a handful of exceptions, investigators who freely disobeyed all the norms set forth by a Bernard or an Osler paid no price for it.

The historical record, particularly as explored by Susan E. Lederer, makes abundantly clear that many investigators demonstrated scant regard for the rights or well-being of subjects. They conducted nontherapeutic research on unknowing or incompetent persons, putting them at risk and causing direct and serious harms. In 1904, a southern physician, Claude Smith, purposefully infected blacks with hookworm to study the transmission of the disease and did not give them the slightest hint as to what he was actually doing. "The patient," Smith stated in his published report, "seemed to have an idea that it was some medicine preparatory to the operation, as nothing was said to him about it."[8] In 1883, George Fitch, resident physician at a Hawaiian leper colony, purposely infected some unknowing eighteen leprosy patients with syphilis to prove the similarities between the two diseases.[9] Another of his colleagues infected relatives of leprosy patients who themselves were free of the disease with the leprosy organism to study transmission. "A splendid field for experimental work was at hand," he candidly wrote, "and stretching all questions of professional ethics, I did not hesitate to avail myself of the opportunities afforded me for testing the inoculability of leprosy."[10]

Some research protocols inflicted such egregious harm on subjects as to earn the condemnation of other investigators. The research by the Italian bacteriologist Giuseppe Sanarelli was a case in point. To prove that he had isolated the bacillus that caused yellow fever, he infected five Montevideo hospital patients with it and claimed (mistakenly) that he had produced the disease in them. William Osler led the attack on the ethics of his research: "To deliberately inject a poison of known high degree of virulency into a human being, unless you obtain that man's sanction, is not ridiculous, it is criminal."[11] In a later and fuller elaboration of this point, Osler explained,

> The limitations of deliberate experimentation upon human beings should be clearly defined. Voluntarily, if with full knowledge, a fellow-creature may submit to certain tests, just as a physician may experiment upon himself. Drugs, the value of which has been carefully tested in animals and are found harmless may be tried on patients, since in this way alone may progress be made, but deliberate experiments such as Sanarelli carried on with cultures of known and tested virulence, and which were followed by nearly fatal illnesses, are simply criminal.[12]

In much these same terms, Osler, and many other colleagues as well, condemned the cancer research that had been conducted by two German surgeons, both of whom took malignant cells from the diseased breast of a patient and injected them into the other, healthy, breast, to study the transmissibility of cancer cells. The *Journal of the American Medical Association* reported the incidents, applauding the subsequent refusal of a French medical academy to discuss the findings because they were obtained in so unethical a fashion. It hoped that "the storm of indignation which has been aroused, shall deter others who mighthave in view, in their zeal for science, [conducted] similar unjustifiable experiments."[13]

The roster of nontherapeutic research on uninformed subjects could be extended almost indefinitely. In 1911, Hideyo Noguchi injected several hundred residents of a New York orphan asylum with an experimental substance, luetin, to learn whether it might serve to indicate the presence of syphilis. Other researchers used orphans to test the efficacy of tuberculin as a vaccine against tuberculosis, as well as to trace the development of such dietary deficiencies as scurvy. So too, researchers subjected black infants at an Atlanta, Georgia, hospital to lumbar punctures without the permission of their parents. One investigator even went so far as to infect an infant with the herpes virus for experimental purposes. As with orphans, prisoners were used as subjects in nontherapeutic and harmful protocols, including one protocol that imposed a diet designed to cause pellagra, and another that injected ameba in order to study the course of dysentery. Finally, investigators in the 1920s used prisoners in San Quentin, California, to study the effects of implants of testicles taken from executed prisoners and rams.[14]

The Disparities Between Ethics and Practice

The research protocols that so flagrantly violated the existing ethical precepts in human experimentation were not carried out covertly or kept hidden from view. To the contrary, the findings were published in the major and widely read medical journals. Nevertheless, the conduct did not incite professional criticism, let alone discipline, except in a handful of cases. To be sure, Osler and several colleagues forcefully condemned some of the protocols described here, including the yellow fever and breast cancer examples. But these were individual reactions and the occasional efforts made to move beyond that to a more official condemnation or censure failed.

Why this professional passivity before these violations of ethics? First, such bodies as the American Medical Association had little authority or organizational standing. Well into the opening decades of the twentieth century, when the profession had managed to impose some standards on medical education and medical licensing, it still did not yet enjoy sufficient status or cohesion to act in concert in the arena of human experimentation. Second, and closely related to its lower status, the profession was unwilling to draw greater attention to ethical misdeeds for fear of arming its critics, particularly the outspoken members of anti-vivisection societies. To concede that some investigators acted irresponsibly was to give ammunition to those who thought that all investigators acted irresponsibly, and thereby subvert the entire research enterprise. Commenting on a recent discussion in the German parliament on research which purposefully infected prostitutes with syphilis, the *Journal of the American Medical Association* joined in the condemnation of the research but, apprehensive about lay reactions, added: "If laymen would divert their attention to charlatans ... the world would be benefited, while these attacks on the regular profession tend to impair the confidence of the public in trained physicians and thus they fall easy prey to unscrupulous quacks."[15] The contention was by no means ill-founded. There was a popular and widespread suspicion about what went on in medical laboratories. Even so, the professional response to the violations was exceptionally timid.

Third, the absence of collective action may reflect the fact that the human subjects put at risk and harmed were almost always marginal to the society. They were poor Southern blacks, or prison inmates, or residents of orphan asylums, themselves vulnerable in all so many ways to abuse but outside the net of public concern. To mount a campaign on their behalf would have been extraordinary, and a reluctance to do so—particularly if it might lower the prestige of medical research—is not altogether surprising. The researchers, in the end, were abusing *other* people's bodies.

Human Experimentation in the United States, 1940-1945

The record that we have explored here provides the context for understanding the conduct of human experimentation in the United States during World War II. The challenges that military needs posed for American medicine were pressing, including how to protect soldiers against malaria, particularly when the Japanese controlled the supply of quinine; how to protect them against influenza, especially in the wake of the 1919 pandemic; and how to protect them against dysentery. Investigators diligently attempted to develop vaccines or antidotes and to these ends, human experimentation was vital. There were few useful animal models available and to compound the difficulties, malaria was not naturally occurring in the United States, dysentery was rare, and influenza unpredictable. For obvious reasons, the diseases could not be researched where they were found, that is, under battlefield conditions. This meant that researchers had to create the very conditions that they had to study. Put more directly, they had to infect subjects with the disease organisms and test their preparations against them for efficacy.

How did the investigators recruit subjects for their research and were they respectful of the norms of consent and do no harm? In the overwhelming majority of cases, the answer is no. The subjects were typically made up of institutionalized mentally disabled persons (suffering from mental illness or mental retardation), institutionalized orphans, and prisoners. None of them were truly capable of giving consent, certainly not the mentally incompetent or the orphaned children, and (although this point has been debated) not convicts deprived of liberty, living in conditions of severe deprivation, and under total state control. Thus, the researchers violated long-standing ethical norms by carrying out non-therapeutic experiments that were dangerous and lacked subjects' consent.

In specific terms, researchers conducted their studies on dysentery in state institutions for the retarded. Indeed, government research grants favored investigators who had "access to various state institutions where facilities for study of dysentery are unexcelled," precisely because hygienic conditions were so primitive. Researchers also carried out their investigations in orphan asylums; the boys at the Ohio Soldiers and Sailors Orphanage, were injected with "killed suspensions for various types of shigella group of bacteria," to see whether the compounds would protect against dysentery. Unfortunately, the preparations proved highly toxic, causing fevers on the average of 104 degrees and leaving the boys exhausted.

The influenza research used subjects residing in state facilities for the retarded, in correctional centers for juvenile offenders, and in state hospitals for the chronic mentally ill. The protocols divided the residents in two—one group received the trial vaccine, the other a placebo, and then both were challenged with influenza virus. The vaccines proved to be of varying efficacy, but all the control group and many of the active agent group contracted high fevers and suffered aches, pains, and debilitation.

The bulk of the malaria research went on in state mental hospitals and prisons. In one series of experiments, psychotic, backward patients were infected with malaria through blood transfusions and then given experimental antimalarial therapies. A psychiatrist was a member of the team, but his function was not to determine the subjects' competency to give consent, but to explain their symptoms to the investigative team.[16]

Thus, the marked disparity between the principles of research ethics and the reality of laboratory practices prior to the issuance of the Nuremberg Code confirms the import of promulgating a formal code. In its absence, individuals cogently and persuasively defined the rules of conduct that should govern human experimentation, but their precepts lacked formal standing or authority. What was so crucial, then, about the Nuremberg Code was not so much its content as its form. Its authors correctly insisted that the guidelines expressed well-known and established values. Its uniqueness lies in the fact that these principles were formally endorsed by a court and presented as a code.

Thus, to understand the history of human experimentation immediately after Nuremberg, it must be remembered that this codification of principles owed little to organized medical bodies. The prosecutors called physicians as witnesses and used them as consultants, but the document stood as the work of judges and its stipulations were realized through a court, not through professional medical bodies. In essence, the initial regulatory effort in human experimentation was external to medicine—which helps to account for both its weaknesses and strengths in the post-World War II period.

The Impact of the Nurmberg Code in the United States, 1947-1966

The externality of the Code to the medical profession helps to explain why Nuremberg exerted so little impact on the conduct of human experimentation in the United States in the immediate aftermath of World War II.[17] Although the Code was certainly known to investigators and government officials, references to it in the medical literature were sporadic and occasional. Even more important, investigators themselves paid little heed to the Code's principles. They continued the practices that had marked research during the period 1941-1945, carrying out harmful nontherapeutic protocols on subjects incapable of giving consent. Accordingly, researchers transplanted cancer cells into demented old men in order to study the body's immune reactions; they fed hepatitis virus to children in institutions for the retarded to analyze the etiology of the disease and try to create a vaccine. They injected patients with radioactive substances to evaluate the dangers of radioactive fallout to the population in the event of an enemy attack. Each of these experiments violated the opening provision of the Nuremberg Code: "The voluntary consent of the human subject is absolutely essential. This means the person involved should have legal capacity to give consent . . . and should have sufficient knowledge and comprehension of the elements of the subject matter involved so as to enable him to make an understanding and enlightened decision." But that maxim did not serve as a barrier to the research.

Why should this have been so? Why did Nuremberg have such limited influence? The answer is not that no one had heard of Nuremberg or read its provisions. Rather, the problem goes deeper. Part of the explanation is that the urgency created by World War II gave way to an urgency created by The War

Against Disease and the Cold War. The search for new knowledge seemed (as it always does?) so important as to justify overriding ethical precepts. In part, too, Americans presumed that the Code had no relevance to them, that is, to real scientists trying to advance the well-being of mankind. Nuremberg was written for Nazis, not for physicians—indeed, many Americans believed, altogether mistakenly, that the perpetrators of the gross misdeeds had not been doctors or authentic investigators, but madmen, political hirelings, or "pseudo-scientists," as Andrew Ivy called them.[18] No less important, however was the fact that the Code stemmed from a judicial process. Composed by lawyers, Nuremberg had no medical imprimatur or professional standing. Since it came from outside medicine, it carried no relevance to medicine.

Inseparable from the question of why researchers for two decades ignored Nuremberg is the issue of defining the ethical standards by which these investigators are rightly judged. The claim is often advanced, usually by physicians but occasionally by others as well, that to fault these investigators for ignoring the principle of consent is to impose the standards of the 1980s on actors and events in the 1950s and '60s, to be guilty of *ex post facto* reasoning. But the glaring weakness of this contention should already be apparent from the recognition, emphasized above, that the relevant principles went back at least to Bernard and Osler, and truly to Hippocrates. Moreover, by the mid-1960s, Nuremberg was not the only collective judgment on ethical research conduct. In 1946, the judicial Council of the American Medical Association promulgated a code of research ethics which required "the voluntary consent of the person."[19] In 1964, the World Medical Association published its Declaration of Helsinki, insisting that subjects be informed of the aims, methods, benefits, and hazards of the research before they participated. A defense of "they knew not what they did" surely seems flimsy.

Nevertheless, the debate on the standards for evaluating the ethics of the 1950s and '60s research continues, most recently and prominently in the public attention devoted to the radiation experiments of this period. In 1994, a journalist in New Mexico, Eileen Welsome, identified by name several persons who had been purposefully injected with radioactive substances and her articles stimulated a flurry of media attention and, in short order, a government investigation spearheaded by a presidential task force. With the cooperation of governmental agencies, most notably the Department of Energy, the task force uncovered an extraordinary number of protocols involving radiation research over the period 1940-1974, including research involving plutonium on ostensibly terminal patients, radioisotope research on children, often mentally disabled, total body irradiation on cancer patients with advanced disease, testes radiation on prisoners, and environmental radiation in various communities.

Courtesy of this investigation, what do we know now that we did not know before? Perhaps the single most important and unexpected finding is just how aware investigators and government officials were of the Nuremberg Code, in particular, and of the principles of research ethics, including informed consent, in general. Despite the minimal coverage given to the Code in the public and medical press, the leadership in the Department of Defense (DOD), the Army and the Navy, and the Atomic Energy Commission (AEC) were fully cognizant of its specific provisions and broader implications. In effect, the ethical standards by which to evaluate the conduct of the researchers were the standards that led up to and were encapsulated in the Nuremberg Code.

The AEC as early as 1947 appreciated that to pass ethical review, human experimentation had, in its own words, to carry an expectation of "therapeutic effect," and had to be "susceptible of proof that, prior to treatment, each individual patient, being in an understanding state of mind, was clearly informed of the nature of the treatment, and its possible effects, and expressed his willingness to receive the treatment." Thus, the AEC documents insisted on the competence and "informed consent" (the AEC actually used the term), of the subjects, and ruled out research with no therapeutic benefit.[20]

When the AEC and the DOD were concerned about the risk to air crews posed by nuclear powered engines and considered using prisoners to test effects of exposure levels, one AEC official, Shields Warren, remarked, "It's not very long since we got through trying Germans for doing exactly the same thing;" another investigator, Joseph Hamilton, warned that the proposal "would have a little of the Buchenwald touch." Indeed, many armed services administrators (especially in the Navy) insisted that human experimentation proceed only with consent from subjects and some investigators did respect the principle.[21]

Nevertheless, and once again, the gap between established principle and deed was substantial. The historical record of radiation research is replete with dispiriting examples of administrators failing to implement the ethics they espoused. Thus, the DOD incorporated the Nuremberg Code into its regulations and then, amazingly, classified the document Top Secret and would not even distribute it within its own network. The AEC banned nontherapeutic research, but did nothing to enforce it within its ranks, including its contract research organizations. Whenever agency lawyers issued recommendations about the desirability of legislation to govern the conduct of human experimentation, other agency officials resisted. Some of them, reminiscent of physicians in the early twentieth century, were fearful of "unfavorable publicity"; others worried that "To commit to writing a policy on human experimentation would focus unnecessary attention on the legal aspects of the subject," and narrow the discretion that researchers' enjoyed.[22]

Perhaps most discouraging, clinical research often sacrificed the well-being of subjects even as researchers and government officials went to great lengths to keep the protocols secret. Thus, Ebb Cade, a fifty-three year old "colored male," who was hospitalized following an auto accident but otherwise enjoyed good health, was injected, without his knowledge or consent, with 5 micrograms of plutonium at the Oak Ridge Army Hospital, as part of a project to study the effects of plutonium on workers. In all, as the presidential task force discovered, "at least twenty-two patients were administered long-lived isotopes in experiments." Nor were these subjects invariably terminally ill, a criterion that in itself is suspect but did carry the rationale of obviating a fear of long-term harmful effects.[23] When the AEC considered the release of some of these research reports, an AEC declassification officer concluded that such a step was unthinkable,

> The document appears to be most dangerous since it describes experiments performed on human subjects, including the actual injection of plutonium into the body. . . . It is unlikely that these tests were made without the consent of the subjects, but no statement is made to that effect and the coldly scientific manner in which the results are tabulated and discussed would have a very poor effect on the public.

There was no evidence for the assumption that consent had been obtained and all of the plutonium protocols violated the AEC ban on non-therapeutic research. As the president's task force rightly concluded: "Concerns about adverse public relations and legal liability do not justify deceiving subjects, their families, and the public."[24]

Thus, in the research conducted as part of the Cold War, as with the research conducted in the war against disease, well-established ethical principles did not restrain or modify investigators' behavior. It was not that they were ignorant of the standards. But in their quest for knowledge—and for grants, prizes, and fame as well—they transgressed them. Again, the subjects who were kept in ignorance and put at risk were almost always members of vulnerable groups. In the 1950s and '60s, as in the 1940s, those who suffered the most harm were mentally disabled or prisoners or minorities. And again, those who broke the codes suffered no adverse professional consequences. To the contrary, professional organizations often praised and rewarded them for their work—as though the importance of their findings overrode violations of research ethics.

Imposing Ethics on Human Experimentation: 1966 to the Present

The critical changes that finally brought ethical standards into the practice of clinical research owe more to an aroused public than a troubled medical profession. Forces external to medicine helped to bridge the persistent and considerable gap that had for so long separated principle from practice. The catalyst was a series of exposés in the 1960s and the early 1970s that made the ethics of human experimentation into headline stories. The behavior of researchers appalled citizens and forced the federal government, specifically, the National Institutes of Health (NIH), to impose new regulations upon clinical research. Put most succinctly, it was scandal that finally brought ethics into the laboratory.

What constitutes a scandal? First, the behavior must be perceived as an offensive to one's moral feelings. Second, it must be committed by someone who is trusted and looked to as an example. Third, it must be making public what had heretofore been a closely guarded secret, known to a small circle of participants but hidden from broader view. In this sense, an ordinary robbery by a thief is a crime not a scandal. To enter the realm of scandal requires that the perpetrator be someone who has been trusted, and the act itself must bring a gasp of surprise and a shudder of revulsion.

It was the 1966 publication by Harvard Medical School professor Henry Beecher, "Ethics and Clinical Research," in the *New England Journal of Medicine,* that cast the record of human experimentation in the mold of scandal. Beecher described in capsule form twenty-two protocols of "dubious ethicality." He named no names and provided no footnotes; the *Journal* had the citations, checked them, and agreed to publish the piece without references. To make certain that the story was not lost—remember that in the 1960s there were few medical journalists and they did not scrutinize the weekly medical journals as closely as they do now—Beecher alerted the popular press to the article, and his disclosures received sustained attention.

The twenty-two protocols were shocking to the conscience. They included the hepatitis experiments on the retarded and the cancer cell experiments on demented old men. They also described military research that withheld known agents of efficacy against rheumatic fever, and research at NIH itself that involved new methods of cardiac catheterization. None of the published articles suggested that the subjects had been informed about the experiments; indeed, many of subjects were incapable of giving consent because of their diminished capacity. When Beecher was asked whether the researchers might have obtained consent but neglected to say so in their publications, he aptly responded: "I have worked on the ward of a large hospital for thirty-five years [and] I know perfectly well that ward patients will not ... volunteer for any such use of themselves for experimental purposes when the hazard may be permanent injury or death."[25]

The twenty-two protocols had appeared in prominent medical journals, including five in the *Journal of Clinical Investigation* and two in the *Journal of the American Medical Association.* They were funded by NIH, by drug companies, and by the armed services, and were carried out at major universities, including Harvard and Case Western Reserve. The protocols, in other words, represented mainstream science at mainstream institutions by mainstream investigators—and no one, until then, had criticized the work.[26]

Why was the public so disturbed by the research? After all, the response might have been more calculating and self-serving. The subjects, after all, were marginal to the society (retarded or senile), the research was very important (curing cancer or creating a vaccine against hepatitis), and by strictly utilitarian criteria, the good that would come might outweigh the injuries imposed. But that was not the position adopted. The popular identification was with the subject, not with investigator.

One reason for this special angle of vision, a looking out onto the world from the vantage point of the underdog, was Nuremberg itself, the significance of the crimes committed by the Nazi doctors. The relative silence that surrounded Nuremberg in the 1950s and early 1960s had finally lifted. Why it took so long for Nuremberg to enter the public consciousness has never been clear—perhaps the events were so traumatic that a kind of psychological repression took hold. But first with the Eichmarm trial, and then with increasing scholarly and media attention thereafter, the events became a more common reference point. It was no longer possible to justify risks and injuries to human subjects on the grounds that the state required answers to pressing medical questions. Even German medicine, once so prestigious, had been corrupted by succumbing to an ideology that state interests trump other considerations.

If Nuremberg was one foundation for new perspectives toward human experimentation, the second was the social awareness that medical advances affected not only the individual patient but society more generally, and given the dimensions of the potential transformations, research had to be reviewed and authorized by someone other than the single investigator. Transplant procedures were one case in point: should this society promote a medical technology that makes the body into a collection of spare and reusable parts? Moreover, physicians themselves were often eager to share responsibilities in decision-making about outcomes and resource allocation. The most noteworthy example was physicians in Seattle establishing a lay kidney dialysis committee (more popularly known as the "Who Shall Live Committee"), to decide who received the lifesaving benefits when the machines were in very short supply. So too, the development of nuclear weapons also encouraged biologists to convene the Asilomar Conference and to delay recombinant DNA research until a broader consensus about its safety was achieved.[27]

Finally, the public reaction was consistent with the sensibilities of the 1960s. This was the decade when the civil rights movement flourished, when most Americans came to view racial discrimination and segregation from the perspective of the disadvantaged minority. When brutish redneck sheriffs threatened peaceful protesters with snarling dogs, Americans identified with the victims, not with the authority figures. And by extension, when investigators took advantage of senility or retardation, Americans identified with the victims, not with the physicians. In all, the 1960s was a moment when the discretionary authority of parents, husbands, principals, wardens, and mental hospital superintendents lost legitimacy, when the rights of children, women, students, prisoners, and mental patients were advanced. In terms of principles, paternalism declined in appeal and autonomy rose. Inevitably, this reorientation entered medicine, promoting change in the conduct of human experimentation.

The impact of these several considerations was substantial because they were easily and quickly led to structural changes. In the United States, more so than in Europe, the federal government was the primary funder of clinical research. The funds were distributed through the grants made by the NIH, and NIH, in turn, was dependent upon Congressional appropriations. Thus, public disapproval of the conduct of human experimentation came to the attention of Congressmen, who then expressed their displeasure to officials at NIH. These officials were acutely sensitive to Congressional reactions, recognizing that disfavor might reduce or cut off appropriations. At the same time, they had ample authority over grantees—whatever requirements NIH incorporated into its grant awards would be readily accepted. In brief, the fact that NIH was at once subordinate to Congress and superordinate to the investigators meant that exposes would affect policy. Put into the framework that we have been analyzing here, for the first time, the governance of human experimentation moved directly into medicine. In this way and in the wake of scandal, ethics and practice finally came together.

The essential regulatory mechanism was the Institutional Review Board (IRB). By federal regulation, all recipients of federal grants must secure IRB approval before conducting research on human subjects.[28] Every grant-receiving institution must establish an IRB, with a membership of no less than five persons, at least one of whom is not be affiliated with the institution. The IRB's mandate is, first, to review clinical research protocols to determine whether the benefits of the proposed research outweigh the risks; second, it must make certain that the investigators have explained all the relevant issues to the subjects and received their informed consent. Although the regulations apply only to federally funded research, many states and the great majority of academic institutions require IRB review for any clinical research performed within their jurisdiction, no matter what the source of funding.

Although IRBs were imposed upon the research community, it is the research community that controls them. To look at the IRB only in terms of its formal structure and organizing principles, it would seem to be a paper tiger. The regulations do not on the whole protect against sloppiness or venality. The power to approve or disapprove research on ethical grounds is granted to a local institutional committee, controlled by members of the same institution that is seeking the funding. It is these insiders that dominate decision making and they are themselves researchers who know that the standards they set for others will come back to affect them as well. Moreover, federal regulations are silent on how the local institution makes appointments to the committee, how long members serve, and on what grounds a member may be dismissed or not reappointed. Hence, it is eminently possible that a member who takes a very hard and uncompromising position on the ethical issues will not be reappointed, and more permissive members will be.

These design features, however, also contribute to the strengths of the IRB. The committee is integral to the institution, its ethical standards incorporated into the ongoing research activities. Since it is colleagues, not outsiders, that make the decisions, a would-be investigator does not want to risk their derision or their rejection. For reasons of self-interest as well as a sensitivity to ethical concerns, they would not dare to propose purposefully infecting retarded inmates of an institution with a virus or radioactive substance, or transplanting cancer cells to senile patients. In the end, the quality of an IRB's work depends inordinately on the conscience and commitment of its members—which is why it appears at once so effective a mechanism to those within a medical institution and so frail a structure to those analyzing it from outside.

Thus, the history of human experimentation makes clear that left to itself, medicine in its collective capacity does not necessarily generate change, even when a sizeable gap separates professed ideals from actual practice. The impetus must come from outside, whether from a court, as with Nuremberg, or from federal regulation, as with the IRB. That said, individual physicians may play a critical role, as witness Andrew Ivy at Nuremberg, and Henry Beecher in the mid-1960s. Even more important, external forces can generate internal conformity to ethical standards, not as thoroughly as some might wish, but, as the IRB itself demonstrates, more successfully than before.

Still, the reluctance of professional medical bodies to move rapidly and effectively to confront challenges to medical ethics is particularly worrisome in light of the challenges that clinical medicine faces today. The rise of managed care and other forms of corporate provider organizations are putting the ethics of clinical practice to new and hard tests; it is uncertain, for example, whether such fundamental principles as the physician's first and final responsibility to the well-being of the patient can survive in a health care system dedicated to generating profits for shareholders and company officers. Clearly the threat requires energetic and principled response from professional medical bodies. In the terms we have been analyzing here, individual declarations of guiding principles will not suffice now, any more than they did when Claude Bernard or William Osler advanced them. What is needed is an assertion of collective responsibility, not singular expressions of dismay. Whether medicine will prove capable of mounting this effort is the question that will dominate medical ethics and medical care in the coming decades.

References

1. Although Nuremberg was not the very first code on human experimenta-

tion promulgated, the two examples usually offered, ironically from Germany (in 1900 and 1931), were so little known as to represent a minor qualification. For a discussion of these codes see Michael A. Grodin, "Historical Origins of the Nuremberg Code," in the book he co-edited with George J. Annas, *The Nazi Doctors and the Nuremberg Code.* New York, Oxford University Press, 1992, pp. 121-144. Some would include the 1946 AMA code, but it was issued very much in response to the Nuremberg trial; see Jay Katz, "The Nuremberg Code and the Nuremberg Trial," *JAMA* 276, 1662-1666, 1996.

2. Quoted in J.P. Bull, "The Historical Development of Clinical Therapeutic Trials," *J Chronic Dis* 10: 222, 1959.
3. For an evaluation of the Nuremberg Code that is, wrongly I believe, dismissive of this history, see Katz, op. cit. #1, 1663. Katz insists that "except for occasional voices to the contrary, little thought had been given to patient consent."
4. Coleman, William. "The Cognitive Basis of the Discipline: Claude Bernard on Physiology," *Isis*, 76: 49-70, 1985. Although Bernard was most interested in establishing physiology as an autonomous discipline and the laboratory as the site of research, his observations on experimentation went beyond animals to man. And his language describing research was consistently aggressive. Experimental medicine was to "dominate nature," "to conquer living nature." (pp. 54, 56).
5. *Transactions Cong. Am. Phys. Surg.*, 7: 1, 7-8, 1907.
6. Withington, C.F. *The Relation of Hospitals to Medical Education.* Boston, Cupples, Uphman, 1886, p. 15.
7. See, for example, the discussion in Gerald L. Geison, *The Private Science of Louis Pasteur* Princeton, NJ, Princeton University Press, 1995, Ch. 9, on the debates as to when it was appropriate to move from animal experiment to clinical trial.
8. Smith, C.A. Uncinariasis in the South, with special reference to mode of infection," *JAMA* 43: 596, 1904.
9. Lederer, S.E. *Subjected to Science: Human Experimentation in America before the Second World War.* New York, Oxford University Press, 1995, pp. 17, 61.
10. St. M. Mouritz, A.A. "Human Inoculation Experiments in Hawaii including Notes of Arning and of Fitch," condensed, arranged and annotated by W. Wade, *International Journal of Leprosy*, 19: 205, 1951
11. Sternberg, George M. "The Bacillus Icteroides (Sanarelli) and Bacillus X (Sternberg)," *Transactions of the Association of American Physicians*, 13: 71, 1898, (discussion of paper by Osler).
12. Op. cit. #9, Lederer, p. 63.
13. Grafting cancer in the human subject," *JAMA* 17: 234, 1891.

14. Op. cit. #9, Lederer, pp. 110-111. For still another experiment on prisoners, this with cholera, see Campbell, Kristine A. "Knots in the Fabric: Richard Pearson Strong and the Bilibid Prison Vaccine Trials, 1905-1906," *Bulletin of the History of Medicine*, 68: 600-638, 1994.
15. Experiments on human beings. *JAMA* 34: 1359 1900.
16. For further details of the American wartime research see, Rothman, David J. *Strangers at the Bedside,* New York, Basic Books, 1991, chapter 2.
17. For an absence of citations to the code in American law, as well as for a discussion of *Bonner v. Moran*, "the only *nontherapeutic* experimentation case decided by a U.S. court before the articulation of the Nuremberg Code," see Annas, George J. "The Nuremberg Code in U.S. Courts: Ethics versus Expediency," in Annas and Grodin, *The Nazi Doctors*, pp. 201-222.
18. Ivy, Andrew. Nazi War crimes of a medical nature. *Fed Bull* 33:133-146 1947. Ivy himself recognized that only some of the investigators fit this category and that the medical profession itself in Germany had been undermined.
19. *JAMA* 132: 1090, 1946.
20. Advisory Committee on Human Radiation Experiments, *Final Report,* October 1995, Washington, D.C. Government Printing Office, 1995, p. 87.
21. Ibid., p. 99.
22. Ibid., pp. 101, 104.
23. Ibid., p. 243.
24. Ibid., pp. 253, 1255, 269.
25. Op. cit. #16, p.75.
26. Ibid., chapter 4.
27. This argument is presented more fully in Edgar, Harold and Rothman, David J., "The IRB and Beyond: Future Challenges to the Ethics of Human Experimentation," *The Milbank Quarterly,* (December, 1995). See also, Rothman and Edgar, "New Rules for New Drugs: The Challenge of AIDS to the Regulatory Process," *The Milbank Quarterly,* Volume 68, Supplement 1, 1990.
28. 45 Code of Federal Regulations 46.101 et. seq.

The Coming of Compassion*

Roger James Bulger

Roger J. Bulger is a graduate of Harvard College (1955) and the Harvard Medical School (1960). He also attended Emmanuel College, Cambridge University (1955-1956). Currently, he is president and CEO of the Association of Academic Health Centers. Prior to joining the association in 1988, for ten years he was president of the University of Texas Health Science Center at Houston, and served as chancellor of the University of Massachusetts Medical Center at Worcester and dean of its medical school for two years previous to that. From 1972-1976, Dr. Bulger was the first executive officer of the Institute of Medicine (IOM) of the National Academy of Sciences. He has held tenured academic posts in internal medicine, community medicine, and public health in four different universities. His laboratory and clinical research was concentrated in the 1960s and 1970s in infectious diseases and the clinical pharmacology of antibiotics.

Over the past thirty years, he has authored numerous articles and essays on medical science and health policy. His books include: *Hippocrates Revisited: A Search for Meaning* (1973), *In Search of the Modern Hippocrates* (1987); *Technology, Bureaucracy and Healing in America: A Post-modern paradigm* (1988); and *The Quest for Mercy: The Forgotten Ingredient in Health Care Reform* (1998).

Dr. Bulger has been a member of numerous national advisory committees and has been chairman of several Institute of Medicine committees. He has been on the board of the Association for Health Services Research since 1991, and served as its president in 1992-1993.

Dr. Bulger has been the recipient of numerous awards and honors, including honorary degrees from Thomas Jefferson Univer-

*Delivered 3 April 1997 at the Twenty-seventh Annual Meeting of the American Osler Society, Williamsburg, Virginia.

sity and the University of Maryland. He is a fellow in the Infectious Disease Society of America, the American College of Internal Medicine, and the Royal College of Physicians. In 1987, he was the Tanner Lecturer at Cambridge University.

It is safe to say that health care in America is changing dramatically. I believe that these changes reflect much of what is happening in the rest of society, a society that is moving from the security of a belief in everlasting material progress (which we have labeled "modernism"), based upon the principles of the Enlightenment as expressed through the successes of the capitalistic, democratic, industrialized nations, to a time of confusion (which we call "post-modernism"), characterized by a decreasing faith in the old principles and with no new governing paradigm readily available to direct us to whatever we may become after the Post-Modern era. The ways of Modernism have brought us many advantages, but they do not provide meaning for one's life or happiness in the living of it. Even the Provost of Yale University, Jaroslav Pellikan, noted classicist, has proclaimed the end of the total reliance upon rationalism and the Enlightenment. "A third intellectual virtue is a sustained, if not significantly chastened, trust in rationality and it's processes. For a variety of reasons, such a trust has been challenged, by an awareness of its fallibility and its limitations. It seems imperative for the university to develop a deepening appreciation for other ways of knowing and thinking which cannot be accommodated easily to the criteria of the Enlightenment and rationalism."[2]

What I propose to discuss briefly in this paper will fall under the following six rubrics: first, what are some of the major forces in the changing health care environment; second, what is health care and who actually delivers it; third, who and what is a healer; fourth, rationing of health care . . . why do we do it . . . what is it . . . and by whom may it be done; fifth, some foundational values underlying our emerging health care efforts; and sixth, what might Hippocrates and Osler think about the implications of all this to the nature of the covenantal relationship between doctors and other health professionals and society. I shall close with a brief sketch of what all of this implies for the education of health professionals in general, and physicians in particular. It is important for me to say at the outset, particularly to an audience as distinguished and knowledgeable as this one, that I fully appreciate the fact that I do not know the answers or all the possible answers to our societal and professional conundrums. If I seem to speak in positive declarative sentences, it is only to simplify the discussion and to provoke reaction, either positive or negative. I do not believe any of us knows these answers with certainty, but I do believe that more and more of those of us who really care about the healing professions and the healing tradition should become involved with thinking about and developing solutions to the questions, changes and problems that beset us as we approach the next millennium.

The Changing Health Care Environment

The dominant myth of modern medical care being those dramatic interventions capable of bringing stricken patients back from the brink of death or severe disability is changing. High science and high technology being administered in a highly paternalistic mode by a specialist physician according to his or her view of the patient's best interests is no longer the preferred mode of operation. As the definition of health care expands beyond the emphasis upon the acute intervention in the curative mode, a new rhetoric of patient-centeredness has taken hold with significant implications for the substantive nature of the delivery and decision-making process. American individualism seems now to be expressing itself poignantly through the patient-autonomy movement as it gives evidence of having become entrenched in our collective thinking about health care. Although physicians can appropriately claim to have always been committed to the patients' best interests, there is more than a subtle difference between, for example, assessing the processes and structure of medical care, as compared to assessing patient outcomes in the quest to determine quality. Patient-centeredness implies a new perspective, even for the most enlightened physicians, requiring them to think beyond what they have done for their patients to what the system has rendered and what the outcome has been for the patient, including his or her satisfaction.

Managed care, especially as expressed through the Health Maintenance Organization has been around for a long time, but its penetration to include the majority of patients is a recent phenomenon. There are those who say that when capitated care reaches the 50 percent mark in a community, its effects upon practice and costs are as though it had a 100 percent penetration. Thus, its sweep to dominance will affect all practitioners and the public has already assumed that all doctors are operating under different economic rules, such that citizens increasingly do not trust that their doctors will act counter to economic incentives in order to advocate the patients' best interests. One can see that the government, the nation's largest purchaser of health care, has shifted its role from that of careful oversight of the care it finances for its citizens to that of a prudent buyer, seeking to cut costs, reduce the national debt and balance the budget.

Behind these shifts are the expanding definition of health care and the ever-growing influence of science and technologic development. The translation of scientific discovery to new technology provides the upbeat hope of every American, that if they are suddenly stricken, ours is a can-do society that will pull out all the stops to achieve a cure. This American characteristic, so often downplayed or underestimated by health economists is what I sometimes refer to as the *epidemiology of hope,* a hope that infuses all of us, even though the high tech stuff is applied at any one moment to a relatively small subset of the population. It is not always so in other societies.

What is Health Care and Who Actually Delivers It?

There is a haunting cartoon that illustrates the heart of what I believe is the central moral issue regarding access to health care which our society has not yet fully confronted. The picture shows an old woman, bent over her cane and clearly disabled, casting a shadow which is larger than she is; the shadow is in the shape of a dollar sign, suggesting that the cost of caring for the patient is larger than the patient and may be becoming more important than the patient. William Blake once wrote the following couplet, "The dog starved at his master's gate/Predicts the ruin of the state."[3] In the post-modern health care context, the couplet might warn us as follows, "The patient suffering unattended at the health system's gate/ Predicts the ruin of the state." In my view, it is how we decide to care for all of our people, and how much of what is available we decide to offer everyone in need of care that will largely define the quality of our society in the years ahead.

If we are increasingly to think in terms of raising our citizens' health status through the equitable distribution of services, we must first agree on the nature of those services. For me, health care is no longer adequately characterized by the curative miracles of modern therapeutic advances; rather it must be thought of as *preventing, curing, and caring.* These three fields of care describe 1) the prevention of disease and the promotion of healthful life styles, governed by the population-based, epidemiological paradigm, and operating within those fields usually included in public health; 2) the curing of disease, governed by the reductionist, biomolecular intellectual paradigm has become almost synonymous with modern American high tech medical care; and 3) the caring for those whose diseases we cannot prevent or cure refers to the care of the chronically ill . . . a growing population whose treatment involves more of what has become known as the bio-psycho-social paradigm than any other. It is too simplistic to think any longer of the first area to be solely in the hands of public health professionals, the second being in the hands of physicians and specialists, and the third being dominated by nurses. In fact, a variety of health professionals are essential to each sector of the health care enterprise. No one profession can claim hegemony over the whole arena; rather it seems axiomatic that what is needed is the delivery of health care via a seamless web of health professional services oriented to the patients' and the public's best interests, rather than each profession's own self-interest. This latter goal would seem to require a degree of coordination, mutual respect, and determination to collaborate, not yet experienced among our leading professions. And yet, more and more expert critics of the emerging systems of care are calling for a new alliance between the health professions and the patients in order to overcome the management imperatives of cutting costs with insufficient regard for quality. Such a new alliance is seen as essential to sustain the balance of cost and quality control, so important for this avaricious sector of our nation's economy.

Who and What is a Healer?

The concept of personal development and working at enhancing one's own personal competencies may be more fully developed in the nursing literature than in medicine, perhaps excluding the psychiatric literature.

A more recent sortie into this area is taken by Carol Taylor of Georgetown University School of Nursing who in her article, *Rethinking Nursing's Basic Competencies,*[4] argues that moral competence should be added as the fourth nursing competency to the more traditional first three, i.e. intellectual, interpersonal, and technical. Taylor asserts, "An increasing tendency to focus primarily on the intellectual and technical competence of nurses is radically redefining nursing and threatening nursing's ability to respond to human need."[5] She describes some practical strategies for developing and maintaining interpersonal competencies among nurses and in effect shows how it could be incorporated into total quality improvement efforts.

William May, in his book, *The Physicians Covenant,*[6] describes five images of the physician as healer. The five images are outlined below; it is not entirely clear whether May thinks that any one healer might adopt any and all of these images at one time or another or whether he thinks that most physicians tend to fall into one of the image categories. Further I am not certain that he sees the fifth image, the physician as teacher, as the final step to maturity as a healer, but I do have that general impression.

Images of the Healer

Fighter?makes war on death and disease
Parent?compassion and benevolence
Technician?technical performance is ultimate
Covenanter?responsibility, service, fidelity
Teacher?assists patient in coping with incurability

Below, I have listed the elements of the progression I believe characterize the evolution of the mature physician, nurse or dentist healer. Against a background of scientific competence, the healer must learn about the richness of human suffering. Such awareness will elicit the felt need to communicate more effectively with patients, to better understand the nature of their personal circumstances and their sense of their pain. Clinical experience soon brings a growing awareness of the need to confront one's own death to whatever extent one can prior to having to face the prospect first hand. All this attunes the clinician to the subtleties of the placebo effect, and the human role in the optimization of the beneficial effects of treatment.

On the Personal Evolution of the Healer[7]

Scientific and technical competence
Understanding suffering
Ability to communicate
Knowledge of the placebo effect and its role in scientific medicine
Coming to terms with death
Expanded roles and three paradigms
Commitment and loyalty

For my part, one of the most extraordinary examples of the therapeutic effect of a human interaction connected with a professional intervention is described by physician-author Fitzhugh Mullan in his autobiographical book, *Vital Signs . . . A Young Doctor's Struggle with Cancer*.[8] As Dr. Mullan tells it, after an almost unbelievable hospital stay of several months duration during which he and his family and care-givers endured a dramatic series of clinical ups and downs, he was at last ready to be discharged home. The morning of his planned discharge, he suddenly became frightened and overwhelmed with a desire to kill himself, a feeling he had never known before. He felt himself on the verge of jumping out of the window, when he informed the nurse of his situation and asked for help. She contacted the psychiatrist on call. The physician who turned up was unknown to Dr. Mullan and appeared to be approximately the same age and level of seniority. The psychiatrist listened to Dr. Mullan's words and then asked only one question, which according to the patient turned the whole situation around. The psychiatrist asked Dr. Mullan, "Do you want me to hold you?" Dr. Mullan broke down and one leaves the scene with the picture of two people holding onto one another, the one gaining the strength necessary to go on to the next laborious stage of recovery from the other strong and healthy person who somehow knew enough to use the right seven words! I personally cannot imagine myself having the skill and sensitivity to decide to say that sort of thing in that situation. The encounter empowered Dr. Mullan to overcome his panic, to go home, and to undertake successfully the rest of his long and laborious return to the full health he now enjoys.

The Placebo Effect . . . a Pill or Operation, a Healing Person or an Institution . . . or all of the Above?

Lain-Entralgo identified the seminal importance of Hippocrates' cleavage of the science and practice of medicine from the intervention of words and the incantations of the shamans who practiced their art at the time.[9] According to Lain-Entralgo,

Hippocrates created the tradition of medicine as the silent art and in so doing led to the separation of medicine from psychiatry, which from then on developed along a separate track. Freud and Jung and their various followers evolved the practice of using words in therapy in ever more arcane and separate venues from the traditional activities of scientific medicine, which in turn had become more closely associated with the reductionist, biomolecular paradigm, which seeks answers to medicine's questions in our molecules and genes. However, recent developments in the neurosciences (neuroendocrinology, neuropharmacology, etc.) have seemed to draw the two areas together.[10,11,12] As the molecular biology of emotion gets addressed more effectively by traditional science, all of us can understand how a person's emotions and beliefs can influence the incredible pharmacy we carry in our own brains. As it becomes clearer in more and more specific situations how a person's neuroendocrinologic or neuropharmacologic response may change under different environmental circumstances, it becomes easier in principle to conceive of the nature of the well-known phenomenon we call "the placebo effect."

The placebo effect is defined as any effect occurring in association with an intervention, but not resulting from any known physiologic function of the intervention. In fact, placebo effects are not always beneficial; such things as major skin rashes and other reactions have been demonstrated to come from non-allergenic placebos in small percentages of subjects. Since Americans have been enamored of technology virtually since our nation's inception, and since our medical profession is known worldwide to be highly interventionist in its utilization of the many new drugs and other techniques constantly being made available, the American patient is being presented, more often than patients in other countries, with new instruments of hope and new venues through which to profit from the combination of the intrinsic effectiveness of the therapy and its associated placebo effect.

In days gone by, physicians were essentially bereft of effective therapies and were left only with the placebo's benefits.[13] Thus, one of France's greatest early nineteenth-century clinicians was quoted as advising the use of all new medicines as often as possible before they cease to become effective. Oliver Wendell Holmes echoed these sentiments when he postulated in the mid-nineteenth century that if all of the medicines in the world were tossed into the sea, ". . . it would be all the better for mankind—and all the worse for the fishes."[14] Finally, in Flexnarian times, L. J. Henderson, the famous twentieth century biochemist said, "Sometime between 1910 and 1912, it became true that for the first time in history, a random patient visiting a random doctor would have had a greater than fifty-fifty chance of profiting from the encounter."[15] Because the placebo effect generally is believed to be in the range of 30 to 50 percent, Henderson can be interpreted as saying that finally in the twentieth century, physicians had the tools to improve upon the placebo effects of their interventions.

Most of us in modern health care practice have tended to minimize the placebo effect and, in fact, have studied it all too infrequently. For example, we have no idea about individual variation in healers' abilities to elicit the placebo effect from patients, although Benson declares that the elicitation of such benefits depends on the degree of trust in the relationship between the healer and the patient.[16,17] It is the conventional wisdom of many experts that the most pervasive and intense placebo effects are elicited when both the patient and therapist believe that the intervention will work, and that benefit is less marked when one or the other doesn't really believe the therapy may work. This point was made in the 1950s when, based upon convincing evidence in experimental animals, a well-known surgeon concluded that tying off the internal mammary artery in patients with compromised coronary artery blood flow would increase the blood flow through the impaired coronaries, such that those with severe angina and cardiac dysfunction might experience symptomatic improvement. He performed surgery on a series of the most severely ill coronary patients and got highly gratifying results, with 85 percent of his patients experiencing dramatic improvement, some even returning to work pain free. As word spread around the country, others performed the surgical procedure with only half to two thirds of patients experiencing improvement, thus justifying a randomized controlled trial in which every other patient had a sham surgical procedure. When it became apparent that the sham surgery produced results comparable to those from the real surgery,[18,19] the trial was stopped, and the surgical procedure was never performed again. It has been said, however, that many of the original patients continued to stand behind the validity of their surgery and of the improvement they enjoyed from it.

In my mind, one of the most powerful, scientifically sound experiments to demonstrate the power of the placebo effect was performed in 1950 by Stewart Wolf, a respected gastroenterologic physiologist who undertook a study of the nausea associated with pregnancy.[20] Each pregnant volunteer subject agreed to have a tube placed in her stomach through which Dr. Wolf could record intragastric pressures. Thus, he recorded the reverse peristalsis in the stomachs of the pregnant women when they reported feeling a wave of nausea. When their stomachs were quiet, he dropped in some Ipekak and measured the immediate and expected reverse peristalsis response along with the reporting of the subjective feeling of being nauseated. Then he told each of them that he was about to deliver through the tube into their stomach a medicine that he believed would stop their nausea. He then waited until the subjects were experiencing the nausea, and then he delivered his medicine, which invariably did in fact stop the nausea and reverse the antiperastaltic movements. The striking fact is that the medicine he delivered was Ipekak, whose pharmacological effect is exactly the opposite of that which the subjects experienced. Dr. Wolf interpreted these results as showing that the patient's trust in him led them to believe that the medicine would work and that their belief caused the *in vivo* secretion of some blocking agent, which prevented the action of Ipekak as well as of whatever molecule caused the naturally occurring nausea of pregnancy. He concluded, "Placebo effects which modify the pharmacologic action to drugs or endow inert agents with potency are not imaginary, but may be associated with measurable changes at the end organs. These effects are at times more potent than the pharmacologic action customarily attributed to the agent."[21]

The previously scientifically tenuous connections between our minds and our bodies are being more fully explicated and explored by a talented array of modem investigators and clinicians.[10,11,12,17] The holistic movement in general speaks to treatment of individual patients by individual therapists. But can we think of beneficial effects occurring to patients on the basis of the trust relationship with groups of people or with institutions? Nurses are well aware of the studies which purport to show that mortality rates in an intensive care unit are lower when the level of communication between doctors and nurses is high rather than low. A most telling illustration of a kind of institutional placebo may be found in the report from a recently published report from a Houston hospital.[22] The study was a randomized control trial involving 616 primiparous women and the care they received during delivery. All patients were cared for by the same team of nurses and doctors, applying the same logic and practice standards to each patient throughout the study. In the control group, 18 percent required a Cesarean section and 55 percent had epidural anesthesia. One of the two experimental groups had only one added feature to the control treatment and environment: a woman who stood in the corner of the delivery room in a white coat with a clipboard and who neither introduced herself nor spoke to anyone during the birthing process. In this group, the rate of Cesarean Section dropped to 13 percent. The second experimental group, differed from the control group only by the presence of a doula, i.e. a woman who introduced herself by name to the patient; who told the patient that she had no expertise in obstetrical care, except for having had a baby herself; and who further told the patient she would stand by her side holding her hand and would be available to talk or answer questions for the patient as needs be. In this third group, the Cesarean section rate fell to 8 percent, and the rate of use of epidural anesthesia dropped to 8 percent. There were analogous progressive improvements in administration of pain medication, neonatal problems, and length of hospital stay for mother and child. These results have been substantiated in other studies done subsequently in other settings.

In the Houston hospital, the hiring of the doula proved to be cost-effective. The importance of studying such interventions by caring figures in different clinical settings has been recently demonstrated by the Robert Wood Johnson Foundation financed study of terminal hospital care, in which the addition of a trained nurse to the care team was evaluated.[23] The function of the nurse was to facilitate physician-patient interaction; to develop patient directives, shorten the period during which patients who die are on mechanical life support; and ultimately to reduce the total cost of terminal hospitalizations for seriously ill older patients. In this randomized trial of patients determined in advance to have a life expectancy of six months or less, a quarter of the patients presenting to the hospital died in the hospital; one-third of those who died lost their savings and/or those of their family in paying for the terminal hospitalization. It was believed that the intervention of a trained nurse would lead to a breaking of the communication log-jam and a reduction of all the worst statistics. The trial to everyone's surprise, proved otherwise, showing that the nurse had a positive effect only upon the patients' families view of the terminal event. Thus, the addition of a person to facilitate communication and caring in this instance produced no measurable benefits sufficient to justify the expenditure of funds necessary to do the job.

Rationing! Why? What? and by Whom? Its Relation to Renewed Efforts to Measure and Assure Quality of Health Services . . .

My intention here is not to engage in an extensive philosophical and ethical analysis of rationing; rather I would like to raise a variety of issues about the way we think about rationing, and its impact on health care as we have defined it. All health professionals understand that we are already rationing health care in the United States as well as in every other country on earth. As the costs escalate and as the technologies proliferate, we shall have to continue dealing with the issue of the most rational and equitable distribution of health care goods to our population. We cannot all have everything that is available.

At the heart of our efforts at rationing (synonym for cost control) in the United States over the past decade or so has been a debate over who shall ration rather than what or how we shall ration.[24,25,26,27] The options for the answer to the issue of who shall ration include the following: the politician and/or government, the manager, the physician or care-giver, the patient, and all of the above. Until recently, the debate has been between choosing the government or the physician. In the background, the characteristic American emphasis upon individual liberty and autonomy has been reflected in a trend towards putting the patient in charge of his other destiny; such a trend is consistent with everything from informed consent to our tendency to supply our people with multiples of goods and services from which they can choose. But patient autonomy appears to have lost ground, as the market revolution to managed and capitated care provided largely by for-profit corporations has gained the initiative. If the nation becomes 50 to 70 percent capitated by the turn of the century, then clearly, rationing will be predominantly in the hands of the manager of the plan in which the patient is enrolled. The implications of that outcome promise to be significant, not only in terms of reduced patients' autonomy and decision-making but in terms of reduced clinical independence for the care-givers. This issue is clearly one which must be followed closely by individual physicians as they seek to inform the public of the implications of changes in the health care system and by the medical profession as it seeks to preserve the essence of physicianhood.

Another way of considering the rationing issue is to ask what may be rationed. In my mind, the answer is three-fold: technology, time and personnel. If the teaching hospital had become the cash-cow which has funded and facilitated the evolution of new technologies and clinical interventions from the findings of basic and applied science, then its conversion from cash-cow to cost-center in a large population-based system runs the risk of so reversing our incentives as to reduce the flow of innovations too drastically to sustain the level of hope our population finds in the high technology system we now have. The most important aspect of our thinking about how to reduce costs associated with technology has to be to devise the best ways to assure that the technologies we do make available are effective and efficient. By doing that assessment better, we can go a long way to controlling costs and keeping as many effective interventions as possible available for all to use.

The second target of the rationer is time. Time is an element that is not so widely appreciated by the public, which generally regards the issue of time in terms of the ease of gaining an appointment and the convenience of the time and place. Capitated care encourages a more efficient use of time, clearly an important dimension to caregivers. A second dimension is much closer to home for care-givers in general, and this dimension is illustrated most dramatically in a study carried out twenty-five years ago at Princeton University's divinity school by John Darley and C. Daniel Batson[28] and published in the *Journal of Personality and Social Psychology.* I refer to this study as "The Parable of the Modern Day Good Samaritan" and have described it in more detail elsewhere.[29]

In essence, a study of the graduating class of divinity students was carried out in which almost every conceivable aspect of the students' personalities, achievements, life, and professional goals were documented in preparation for the unsuspected experimental defining moment, which occurred for each of them one December day. The group had been divided in two, with half receiving an assignment to write a paper on the Parable of the Good Samaritan and the other half receiving an assignment to write a paper on another passage from the Bible not overlapping substantively with the Parable. Each student was assigned a faculty member that day, and had a one-on-one interview concerning the nature of the paper the student had written to satisfy the assignment. During the interview, a messenger arrived with the news that a visitor wanted to see the student in the administration building concerning a job for the next year. Each student was told one of three things: to run over there posthaste because time was so short; to go over with all deliberate speed to make the appointed time; or to leave now but take your time because the visitor could not see the student for some twenty or thirty minutes.

On the way to the administration building, each student passed a person lying in tatters on the ground, moaning and groaning, in a way analogous to the way we all envision was the case when the original Samaritan encountered his person in need. The sufferer in this case however was a trained observer who noted who stopped, how long they stopped, and what they did when they stopped. In brief summary, when all the data was analyzed, the only variable that had a relationship to who stopped and what they did when they stopped was how much time the individual had.

The conclusion has to be that even the best educated and the most intellectually prepared to consider compassion, and those whose characters most dispose them to be compassionate, cannot show compassion if they do not have enough time. It takes time to listen to a patient and to build the trust necessary to empower the patient's own healing capacities. It is easy to see how an efficient scheduling of patients might so reduce the time and trust that the placebo effect is reduced, and patient outcomes are less positive than they otherwise might have been.

The third target for the rationer will be personnel or payroll and in some cases this may be related to the time element discussed above. For example, in the United Kingdom, Michael Ashley-Miller[30] recently reported that a consulting group to a British hospital, seeking to reduce costs, concluded that the hospital's financial target could be met by reducing the nursing staff by 350 people. The remaining nurses could pick up the tasks of those who had been released if they simply stopped talking to the patients! Apparently the consultants in that case failed to understand why the nursing staff is the heart and soul of the hospital.

The forces requiring cost control and efficiency in delivery are the same as those that lead to whatever venues our society uses to ration; but these forces also should encourage health professions' educators to more effectively and aggressively prepare students to work collaboratively in teams with other health professionals, giving new credence to the concept behind the multiprofessional academic health center.

Because of the cost problems, there is a tendency to see all evaluative research, whether it focuses on structure, process or outcomes, as thinly veiled efforts to cut expenses. Our goal must be to transcend the interest in cost control, to focus instead on value for dollars spent and on the overall quality of the enterprise. Thus, continuous quality improvement is a movement we must truly embrace; it must become more than a rhetorical device used to convince outsiders that we understand the modern management world; it needs to become a central focus of all our efforts if we are to help the public decide that rationing must not include the withholding of truly effective interventions and services from the people. Quality of care must come to be seen in terms of overall process and outcome for the patient. It must be perceived as more than technical competence, and as the net result of the work of all people and institutions that provide services in the attempt to prevent and cure disease and to minimize suffering. Seen in this way, our struggle for high quality will never end.

Some Foundational Values for any American Health Care System . . . a Slightly Different List

Over the past three years, I have had, for the first time since I was seven years old, the necessity (opportunity?) of engaging the modern American, high technology health care system as a patient suffering from a life-threatening illness. In the course of working through that experience and processing its meaning with other information from the worlds I usually have inhabited as a physician, health professions educator and policy wonk, I have developed a slightly different list of foundational values than the one I had before I got sick (Happily by the way, I'm better, no longer deserve sympathy, and will likely cross the bar ultimately from plain old age).

The first three on my list of foundational values have been discussed or alluded to in this essay. They are justice, patient autonomy, and hope. Most of us agree that we would prefer an equitable distribution of effective health care across the entire population. Most of us would also agree that the trend towards patient autonomy is an important and major contribution of our culture to health services in general; and we would certainly not want to remove patient decision-making from our agenda. Hope may not be so widely embraced as the first two. By hope, I mean the hope we all have that if serious illness or disease or disability strikes us as individuals, that we would have a chance to receive the care and interventions that might restore us to health or to a decent quality of life. The interests of the group do not always coincide with those of the individual; but the social value of hope links heroic individual interventions to the concerns of everyone. It is hard to put a market value on hope; although without it, no one would really want to pay very much for health care.

It is in presenting the fourth value that I feel uncertain as to its general acceptability. Clearly, this fourth value dented my consciousness only as a result of my recent illness and my attempts to consider what this gigantic jigsaw puzzle of specialists, services, institutions, technologies, and human beings really meant. The concept first hit me when I was reading something autobiographical by Thomas Merton. Merton[31] gained fame as the modern Trappist Monk, who left a secular life as writer, artist, and teacher to find meaning in the development of his spiritual life outside the mainstream of the modern world. He said, in an attempt to summarize the lessons he had learned during his long sojourn in the monastery, the following: that the entire meaning of his spiritual life was bound up in the words of the ritual the Trappists have used for centuries when a new monk enters. They are as follows, Questioner: "What do you ask?" Supplicant Monk, "I ask the Mercy of God and of the Order."

I puzzled over that answer of Merton's, which seemed vacuous and rather bland to me until I read elsewhere in another context that the word mercy actually means, the enveloping love of the womb. When I applied that meaning to Merton's answer, it became a much richer answer, and made even more sense to me when I turned it into a dialogue between a seriously ill or damaged patient in our modern society. In such a situation, the dialogue might go as follows: Questioner, "What do you ask?" The patient answers, "I ask the mercy of the health care providers and of the community in which I live."

The more I reflected on my own interaction as a patient with the health care system, this dialogue rings true and I therefore, include on my list of foundational American values for our health care system the value of mercy. How you sell it, how you price it, how you provide for it in the organized delivery system's expense column are all difficult questions. Nonetheless, I find it to be a key societal value, about which we should be talking more. I am equally certain that nursing knows more about this value than any of the other professions, and that we must look to nurses to teach us and the public about it. As far as I, a former patient, am concerned, if health care is the game, mercy or compassion is its name.

Hippocrates and Osler Revisited

Hopefully, by now, the reader will see the rationale behind my insistence upon the health care team, and the inherent deduction that our separate covenantal oaths should add something in common to all about the importance of interprofessional collaboration. Each of the major health professions shares with the Hippocratic oath an avowal to competence, to compassion and to commitment; to these three there should be in my view a fourth "c" added, collaboration. A multiprofessional group has developed the following proposed amendment in common to each of the major professions' oath,

> As a health professional dedicated to enhancing the health care status and well-being of individuals and communities, I pledge collaboration with all of my health professional colleagues similarly committed, and promise, should tensions or conflicts of interests arise, to place patient and public interests above the perceived self-interests of my individual profession.

It may be of some interest that nursing, dentistry, pharmacy and allied health professional deans have all agreed, but allopathic and osteopathic medicine deans have not on the grounds that their oaths already say as much! It seems there is a way to go before the concept of teamwork in the patients' interest is fully accepted.

I sometimes muse about Hippocrates and the followers he gathered under that plane tree on Cos. If he were to gather scientific healers around him again today in our context, would he restrict his circle to physicians and if so would he include all physicians, even those doing epidemiology or laboratory investigation? Would he include clinicians of various stripes with direct patient service as their common bond? Would this grouping then include physicians, nurse practitioners, nurse midwives, dentists, clinical psychologists, physical therapists and physicians' assistants? Would he adapt to the patient-centered focus, placing it ahead of short-term perceived professional issues? Where would Osler be on these issues? Osler, the science-based clinician who spent many hours visiting a terminally ill child, talking with him in the presence sometimes of the parents about death and separation, with seeming success in relieving some of the agony and pain of the passing for patient and family alike, would it seems to me take great pains, were he operating in our post-modern condition, to do that sort of thing when he could, but to be certain that someone from the therapeutic team did so.

Educational Implications

If we are to sustain the millennia-old tradition of the therapeutic person or professional, we shall have to be more explicit about how we educate for this result. Our physician education has of necessity been oriented to the never-ending quest for technical competence. In my own mind, there is a second educational path (see above, on the personal evolution of the healer), which goes on in parallel, but over a different time course, both in and out of the formal educational processes, than does the education for technical competence. This second pathway involves the personal growth of the care-giver, includes some study and skill acquisition (as in interpersonal communication skills), but goes far beyond that to include every day experiences, values, character, service-orientation, involving also interactions with the arts, anthropology and a curiosity about the community with which one is involved. Clearly, my idea of the second path is not everyone's, but equally clearly it seems to me, all who pretend to be serious medical educators should be thinking about these matters seriously and trying to see how they can include aspects in the formal and informal curricula, that constitute undergraduate and postgraduate medical education.

For example, societal values undergirding the health care system (my list includes *justice, autonomy, hope, and mercy)* and foundational professional values (my list includes *competence, compassion, commitment, and collaboration)* should be expressed and pointed out within the formal medical curriculum and should also form a series of prisms through which evaluative efforts are viewed. In summary, we need to remember that the continuum of health care represents a vast and culturally important societal expression of mercy and compassion, from all of us to each of us. As professionals, we have a crucial role in this entire enterprise. Our value rests not only in our collective competencies to diagnose, to prevent and to cure, but in our commitment to caring, to seeing the patient through to a decent end and to persistently demanding quality services from ourselves, from our filial health professions partners and from the managers. As physicians, we are the natural leaders of the enterprise and although the time is past when we can, simply assume that position on the basis of our status, we can with Osler's equanimity, competence and humanity, earn that position.

References

1. Bulger, R.J. Old wine in new bottles—nursing in the 21st century. *J Professional Nursing* 12: 338-348, 1996. This essay has its roots in and shares much of its substance with the John P. McGovern Award Lecture presented at the American Association of Colleges of Nursing's annual meeting on 22 October, 1995.
2. Pellikan, J. 1992.
3. Blake, W. "Auquires of Innocence," quoted in Bartlett, J. *Familiar Quotations . . .* 13th ed. Boston, Little, Brown, 1955, p. 388.
4. Taylor, C. Rethinking nursing's basic competencies. *J Nursing Care Quality* 9: 1-13, 1995.
5. Ibid., p. 5.
6. May, W. *The Physician's Covenant*. Philadelphia, Westminister Press, 1983.
7. Bulger, R.J. *The Quest for Mercy: The Forgotten Ingredient in Health Care Reform.* Charlottesville, VA, Carden Jennings, 1998.
8. Mullan, F. *Vital Sign?A Young Doctor's Struggle with Cancer*. New York, Farrar, Straus & Giroux, 1975.
9. Lain-Entralgo, P. *The Therapy of the Word in Classical Antiquity.* New Haven, CT, Yale University Press, 1970.
10. Kiecolt-Glaser, J.K. and Glaser, R. Psychological influences on immunity. *Psychosomatics* 27: 621-624, 1986.
11. Pert, C.B., Ruff, M.R., Weber, R.J. and Herkenham, M. Neuropeptides and their receptors: A psychosomatic network. *J Immunology* 135 (Suppl): 820s—826s, 1985.
12. Institute of Medicine of the National Academy of Sciences. *A Research Briefing: Behavioral Influences on the Endocrine and Immune Systems.* Washington, DC, National Academy Press, 1989.
13. Bulger, R.J. The demise of the placebo effect in the practice of scientific medicine—A natural progression or an undesirable aberration? *Trans Am Climatological Assoc* 102: 285-293, 1991.
14. Holmes, O.W. Address, Massachusetts Medical Society, (30 May 1860) quoted in Bartlett, J., *Familiar Quotations,* Boston, Little, Brown, 1995, p. 536 .
15. Op. cit., #13, Bulger, p. 285.
16. Benson, H. and Epstein, M.D. The placebo effect: A neglected asset in the care of patients. *JAMA* 232: 1225, 1975.

17. Benson, H. & McCallie, D.P. Angina pectoris and the placebo effect. *N Engl J Med* 300: 1424, 1979.
18. Beecher, H.K. Surgery as placebo: A quantitative study of bias. *JAMA* 176: 1102-1107, 1961.
19. Cobb, L.A., Thomas, G.I., Dillard, D.H., Merendino, K.A. and Bruce, R.A. An evaluation of internal mammary artery ligation by double blind technic. *N Engl J Med* 260: 1115-1118, 1959.
20. Wolf, S. Effects of suggestion and conditioning on the action of chemical agents in human subjects: The pharmacology of placebos. *J Clin Invest* 29: 100-109, 1950.
21. Ibid., p. 104.
22. Kennell, J., Klaus, M., McGrath, S., Robertson, S. and Hinkley, C. Continuous emotional support during labor in a U.S. hospital. *JAMA* 265: 2197-2201, 1991.
23. Support Principal Investigators. A controlled trial to improve care for seriously ill hospitalized patients. *JAMA* 374: 1591-1599, 1995.
24. Bulger, R.J. *Technology, Bureaucracy, and Healing in America: A Post-modern Paradigm*. Iowa City, University of Iowa Press, 1988.
25. Eddy, D.M. Rationing by patient choice. *JAMA* 265: 105-108, 1991.
26. Reiser, S.J. Consumer competence and the reform of American health care. *JAMA* 267: 1511-1516, 1991.
27. Wennberg, J.E. *Regional variations and outcomes research.* Presented at the Association of Academic Health Centers Annual Meeting, Tucson, AZ, 1989.
28. Darley, J.M. and Batson, D.D. From Jerusalem to Jemcho: A study of situational and dispositional variables in helping behavior: *Personality and Social Psychiatry* 27: 100-108, 1973.
29. Bulger, R.J. Tragic choices and the modern-day good samaritan. *The Washington Post,* Health Section, July 5: p. l, 1988.
30. Ashley-Miller, M. United Kingdom Issues. The Health Workforce: Power, Politics, and Policy. Washington, DC, Association of Academic Health Centers, 1996.
31. Merton, T. *The Seven Story Mountain*. New York, Harcourt, 1948.

Why We Go Back to Hippocrates*

Paul Potter

Paul Potter is Jason A. Hannah Professor, and Chairman of the Department of History of Medicine at the University of Western Ontario in London, Ontario, Canada.

He graduated M.D., C.M. from McGill University in 1968. He then turned to full-time study of the Classics, first at McMaster University in his native city of Hamilton, Ontario, and then at Kiel, Germany, where he was awarded the D.Phil. in 1973 for his dissertation on the Hippocratic treatise *Diseases III.* Since that time he has been a member of the Faculty of Medicine at the University of Western Ontario, where he has taught a wide variety of students and carried on research in several areas of Medical History.

Dr. Potter's primary research commitment has been to the ancient Greek medical writings, in particular those transmitted under the name of Hippocrates of Cos. His editions and translations have appeared in the *Corpus Medicorum Graecorum* (1980), and the *Loeb Classical Library* (1988-1995).

*Delivered 6 May 1998 at the Twenty-eighth Annual Meeting of the American Osler Society, Toronto, Ontario.

Life is short, the art is long.

Hippocrates

With the name Hippocrates, Western medicine connects its earliest and most formative phase, the ancient Greek roots from which it has continued to draw its nourishment, both technical and professional, for almost two and a half millennia. In the pages that follow, I will attempt to illustrate just what it is we owe to this remarkable era, and why its influence has been, and must continue to be, so fundamental for us.

But before I turn to the writings attributed to Hippocrates themselves, let me first say a few words about the Greek world into which Hippocrates was born, some time around 460 BC, and in which he grew up. Long before his medical instruction began, Hippocrates' world view would have been shaped by two powerful forces. These were the tradition of storytelling embodied in the Homeric Epics, the *Iliad* and the *Odyssey,* which dated back several centuries by his time; and the habit of uninhibited questioning about the universe and man's place in it, which had begun with philosophers like Thales and Xenophanes in the sixth century, and which by the middle of the fifth century had come to pervade every aspect of Greek thought and expression, from the plastic arts to politics, from poetry to drama, from astronomy to architecture.

The Homeric poems formed the centerpiece and touchstone of all Greek education, linguistic, political, and religious. The heroes, if not exactly models to live by, did incorporate the virtues and weaknesses which characterize human life at its deepest level. The gods, if no better than they should be in their personal behavior, did present a regulatory framework within which the events of individual and collective human life might be connected and explained. It was the world of Achilles and Odysseus, together with the language itself of the poems, which gave Greek culture its identity, and from which every specific human activity took its beginning. About the healer (*iatros,* derived from the verb *iaomai* "I heal") and his art, Homer's few explicit statements confirm little more than that by the eighth century BC healing was a highly valued skill (*Iliad* 11, 514), and that its practitioners belonged to the class of itinerant experts that included, as well, the seer, the bard and the architect (*Odyssey* 17, 383-384).

Perhaps most influential in Hippocrates' formation as a future physician were two general features of Homeric thought. First, an unbounded enthusiasm for the details of the sensible world, which encouraged the accurate observation and description of everything from stars and clouds to plants and animals, to city walls and works of art, all viewed with a kind of wonder (*thauma idesthai*) not untinged with religious awe. When Odysseus builds a raft, we follow him from the felling of the trees to his preparation of its last technical fixture (*Odyssey* 5, 233-242), when a warrior is wounded, the missile's course is followed (e.g. "the spear . . . struck Sarpedon even where the diaphragm clasps the beating heart"

[*Iliad* 16, 480-481]) and its effects explained (e.g. ". . . right through the tender neck went the point, yet the bronze-weighted ashen spear broke not through the windpipe, so that Hector could yet speak" [*Iliad* 22, 328]). Attention to observed detail—even for its own sake—then, is a basic Greek cultural trait.

The second way of thinking inherent in the Epics which has a special significance for medicine—an art in which the establishment of causal links has always presented particular difficulties—is a kind of pre-Aristotelian causality. As the action of the poems unfolds, the growth of the present out of the past and towards the future is frequently explained, but not, however, always on the same level. Each Homeric hero has from the moment of his birth a pre-established Fate which determines the main course of his life, and ultimately his death. But each person also has a clearly articulated individual character or personality which informs his acts and gives them a unity and consistency. The Homeric individual's thoughts and actions follow naturally from this character. Thirdly, there are the gods sitting on Mount Olympus who play an active role in influencing the actions and sufferings of their human favorites and/or enemies by specific interventions on land and sea. Now when any event occurs in the poems—for example, when in book twenty-two of the *Iliad* Hector goes forth to meet Achilles in battle and thereby meets his doom—it can be and often is explained on one, two, or even all of the three levels described: a) Although Hector has been told by the dying Patroclus that he himself will fall by the hand of Achilles (16, 852-854), his patriotism for Troy and his momentary feeling of personal prowess overcome his better judgement, leading him to *decide* to face Achilles (22, 99-130); b) when Zeus weighs the lots of Hector and Achilles, Hector's fatal day sinks to Hades (22, 208ff.); c) as the duel progresses, Apollo, after helping Hector once, suddenly deserts him, while Athena appears as helper at Achilles' side (22, 216ff.). This sophisticated poetic device often leads to contradictory statements by the poet about the hierarchy of these causes. Occasionally, it would seem that a god, in particular Zeus, might be able to override Fate, or at least to postpone what is fated (*Iliad* 16, 852-854), while in the general case Fate is clearly held to be supreme. Sometimes a hero's character leads apparently by itself to his destruction, at other times his death seems to be determined by his Fate alone, or by the direct act of a god; and so forth. Hippocrates, like us, faced many medical cases in which the competing causalities of a specific preceding event, life-style in general (*diaite,* in Greek), and environmental or epidemiological factors all seemed to be implicated, but where the interactions between the discrete causal chains of events leading to the same disease occurrence were indeterminable. That the Hippocratic writers are willing to describe illnesses unbiasedly, to hypothesize about their possible causes on many levels, but ultimately to leave the question of causal hierarchy open, is a Homeric heritage.

This general interest in natural phenomena and their causes displayed in the Homeric writings evolved, by the sixth century BC, in such a way that the actions of the gods—especially the anthropomorphic Homeric gods—in the world came to be regarded as merely a poetic or metaphorical expression for processes henceforth to be explained in terms of physical (*physis* in Greek means "nature") abstractions: number, form, material, space, the forces of attraction, repulsion, mixing, separation, et cetera. This new turn of mind first appeared in the Greek city-states along the Ionian coast of Asia Minor (the island of Cos, Hippocrates' birthplace lies just off this coast), especially Miletus and Ephesus, as well as in several Greek colonies of southern Italy such as Agrigentum and Croton.

These new thinkers sought to discover through observation and/or speculation the regular, permanent entities "behind" the inconstant, everchanging appearances of the observed world. Some put forward the theory that some single indestructible material "beginning" (*arche*) underlay everything: water (Thales), air (Anaximenes), fire (Heraclitus), or some indeterminate element, *apeiron* (Anaximander); for others it was a combination of the four elements, earth, air, fire and water (Empedocles) exchanging places within a "full" universe, or again numberless finite particles (*atomoi*) ricocheting off one another in the void (Democritus), that explained the world. Other materialist thinkers asked questions such as how a baby is able to convert its sole nourishment, milk, into all the tissues of its body (*Anaxagoras*), or how a specific plant's roots "know" which elements to extract from the soil to give it its particular essence.

Numbers as determinants of reality were also closely studied. Pythagoras analyzed musical sounds mathematically according to the relative lengths of lyre-string that produced them, expressing the notes of the scale as ratios. Empedocles, combining the material with the numerical, gave us our first—admittedly highly speculative—chemical formula: bone is four parts fire, two parts earth, and two parts water (Fragment 96).

This philosophical study of nature reached its acme just at the time of Hippocrates' youth. Secondary education in fifth century Greece was acquired by listening to the public lectures delivered by various of these traveling "sophists" in the town gymnasium, or even by attaching oneself to one of them for a fee, with whom one then traveled about Hellas for a number of years learning the master's precepts. This was the immediate intellectual background against which the writings of the Hippocratic Collection were written, in whose terms their theoretical discussions are framed.

The body of approximately seventy writings, ranging in length from one page, e.g. the *Oath,* to several hundred pages, e.g. *Diseases of Women* 1-3, that constitute the Hippocratic Collection date in the main—as far as scholars can tell—from Hippocrates' lifetime, or a little later, from about 440-360 BC. The actual relationship of the individual treatises which vary considerably in their medical theories, their areas of interest, and their literary form, to the historical Hippocrates, to whom both Plato (427-349) and Aristotle (384-322) refer as a leading physician of the fifth century, has been discussed since at least the first century AD (cf.

Erotianus, *On Hippocratic Words,* preface), probably even much earlier, without any generally agreed upon conclusions being reached. The possibility that all seventy writings are by Hippocrates is definitely excluded by their diversity alone; that none are by Hippocrates, who according to Plato had established a wide reputation for his medical theories and practice by about 433 BC (*Protagoras* 311b; cf. *Phaedrus* 270c-e), seems almost equally improbable. Let us for today leave the debate about specific cases to the historical scholars, and work on the principle that the majority of the Collection, which does indeed tend rather towards a unity of medical and surgical viewpoint than to the contrary, represents medicine as Hippocrates taught and practiced it, and call this Hippocratic medicine.

In what follows I shall present a number of Hippocratic passages—some well known, others less so—that seem to me to illustrate their medicine's main features; not surprisingly, much of what appears here has palpable intellectual connections to the Homeric and early philosophic thought mentioned above. As five defining features of this medicine, let us examine the headings: 1) clinical observation; 2) theoretical reasoning; 3) the use of experience and experiment; 4) medicine's intermediate position between a science and an art; 5) the art of therapy.

William Osler, in his *Principles and Practice of Medicine* (1892), refers explicitly to Hippocratic texts fourteen times, many of them containing clinical observations. Perhaps most famous among these descriptions are the *facies hippocratica* of the cachexic patient from *Prognostic* 2 (Osler, p. 464), the clubbed or Hippocratic fingers associated with disease of the chest from *Internal Affections 10 (*pp. 230 and 992), the "winged scapulae" of consumption from *Epidemics* 3, 14 (pp. 192 and 225), and the principal features of the epileptic attack detailed in *Sacred Disease 10* (p. 951). This habit of careful observation among the Hippocratic writers upon which Osler draws includes, besides a very considerable number of signs and symptoms, both longitudinal studies seeking to relate hereclity, habits, and disease (cf. Osler quoting on gout from *Prorrhetic 2* 8, p. 287, and on epilepsy from *Prorrhetic 2* 9, p. 954), and community studies attempting to bring the morbidity and mortality observed in individual communities into relationship with their geographical position, their water supplies, and the winds to which they are subject (*Airs, Waters, Places*), and recording the annual health status of specific places in specific years (*Epidemics* 1 and 3). As an example of a general disease description, I quote the first recorded account of mumps:

Many had swellings beside one ear, or both ears, in most cases unattended with fever, so that confinement to bed was unnecessary. In some cases there was a slight heat, but in all the swellings subsided without causing harm; in no case was there suppuration such as attends swellings of other origin. This was the character of them: flabby, big, spreading, with neither inflammation nor pain; in every case they disappeared without a sign. The sufferers were youths, young men, and men in their prime, usually those who frequented the wrestling school and gymnasia; few women were attacked. Many had dry coughs which brought up nothing when they coughed, but their voices were hoarse. Soon after, though in some cases after some time, painful inflammations occurred either in one testicle or in both, sometimes accompanied with fever, in other cases not: usually they caused much suffering. (*Epidemics* 1, 1)

It was observations like these which, coupled with clinical reasoning, led to the general theory of epidemic disease causation in men and animals put forward in *Breaths 6:*

Now epidemic fevers occur this way because all men inhale the same air; and when the same air has been taken up by the same kind of bodies, the same fevers result. . . . So whenever the air has been infected with pollutions (miasmas) that are hostile to the human body, men will become ill, but when the air becomes unsuitable for some other species of animals, then they will become ill.

This type of reasoning direct from the observed features of disease was often extended to include various semi-hypothetical bodily substances and processes in a way analogous to the "chemical" reasoning of the philosophers mentioned above. Most frequently, reference was made to certain fluid components of the body—either the pair phlegm and bile, or, by the addition of blood and black bile, the canonical four humours, which mirror Empedocles' system of the four elements. It was changes in these fluids, explained according to generally held principles involving rarefaction and condensation, warmth and cold, attraction towards an empty space, and the tendencies of heavy things to move downwards and of light things to move upwards, that were held to lead—often directly and naively—to observed signs and symptoms. For instance,

> When the head becomes overheated, the patient passes much urine; for the phlegm in the head melts, and, as it melts, some runs to the nostrils, some to the mouth, and some through the vessels that lead to the genital parts: when it arrives in these parts, the patient urinates fre quently, and strangury develops. (*Diseases* 2, 1)

Sciatica usually arises as follows: if a person is exposed for a long time to the sun, and his hip-joints become heated, the moisture in them is dried up by the burning heat. My proof (*tekmerion*) that the moisture is dried up and congealed is this: the patient cannot turn and move his joints, because of the pain in them, and because his vertebrae have become fixed. (*Internal Affections* 51)

From these cases, and many more like them, the important roles that observation of, and reasoning about, naturally occurring disease phenomena play at the centre of Hippocratic medicine are evident. But what about the experiment, the artificially created situation from which evidence can be gathered to test a specific hypothesis? In fact, examples—albeit infrequent and varying in their degrees of perfection—of the experimental method are found in both the clinical and the theoretical writings of the Collection.

These experiments are included in the general category of evidence called a sign (*semeion*), proof (*tekmerion*), or witness (*martyrion*), of which a clinical example is quoted above in an account of sciatica. Presumably because the experimental method was just in the process of being formulated, our writers use it with a considerable degree of freedom, not to say looseness. The hypotheses being tested are often left implicit, quantities are rarely measured, the conclusions drawn are frequently not logically justified from the evidence—in fact even whether the experiment being described was actually carried out or remained in the "thought-experiment" stage usually remains unsure.

A number of clinical tests clearly represent simple experiments, e.g.,

> [In cases of empyema] soak a piece of fine linen in warm, moist, finely ground clay; then wrap this around the patient's chest, and, wherever it first dries, that is where you must cauterize or incise, as close to the diaphragm as possible, but sparing the diaphragm itself. (*Diseases* 3 16)

> . . . if you cannot otherwise distinguish by inspection whether the skull is fractured or contused or even both, then you must apply to the bone a very black solution and anoint the wound with the same. . . . Next day, after opening and cleaning the wound, scrape further, and, if it is not sound but fractured and contused, the rest of the bone after scraping will be white, but the fracture and the contusion will have absorbed the solution and will appear black in the white bone. (*Wounds in the Head* 14)

> This is how you can tell he is blind: if you bring your finger near his eye, he does not blink. (*Internal Affections* 48)

> Pinch the patient with three fingers: if he feels it, his condition is hysterical, if not, his condition is spastic. (*Regimen in Acute Diseases* [*Appendix*] 68)

In the theoretical discussions of the Collection, over a dozen experiments are described, most seriously flawed methodologically in the ways noted above. The author of the embryological treatise *On the Nature of the Child,* however, puts forward an experiment with a much more modern ring.

> If you take twenty or more eggs and place them to hatch under two or more hens, and on each day, starting from the second right up to the day on which the egg is hatched, you take one egg, break it open and examine it, you will find everything as I have described it. (Chapter 29)

A physical experiment involving actual measurements is cited in *Airs, Waters, Places* 8 as proof that water on freezing loses a part of its material essence,

> Pour by measure, in winter, water into a vessel and set it in the open, where it will freeze best; then on the next day bring it under cover, where the ice will melt best; if when it is melted you measure the water again, you will find it much decreased in amount.

The unreserved confidence with which the Hippocratic writers expound their scientific views based in observation, reasoning, and to a limited degree experimentation reflects a professional maturity which no doubt grew out of generations, probably centuries of collected experience,

> Medicine has long had all its means to hand, and has discovered both a principle and a method, through which the discoveries made during a long period are many and excellent; and what remains will be discovered if the inquirer is competent and conducts his researches with knowledge of the discoveries already made, and makes them his starting point. But anyone who, casting aside and rejecting all these means, attempts to conduct research in any other way or after another fashion, and asserts he has found anything out, both deceives others and is deceived himself. (*Ancient Medicine* 2)

But if medicine's method is as secure as this writer claims, why is medical practice so difficult, a fact repeatedly stressed throughout the Collection in passages such as the one from *Aphorisms* 1 that Osler chose for the motto of the *Principles and Practice:* "experience is fallacious, judgement difficult?" The answer to this question lay for the ancients in medicine's middle position between a science and an art. Whereas a pure science such as geometry is a system of reasoning consistent and complete in itself, apart from the every day world, and may thus be reduced to a totally rational basis, medicine as practice most definitely belongs to the world of appearances. The physician is called upon to deal with diseases whose causes may be partly elucidated by his science, but whose manifestations in the individual patient are subject to an almost infinite set of variables,

> Among persons that have these and similar diseases, a man differs from a woman in the ease or difficulty with which he recovers, a younger man differs from an older man, and a younger woman differs from an older woman; additional factors are the season in which they have fallen ill, and whether or not their disease has followed from another disease. Besides, one affection differs from another, being greater or less, one

> body from another, and one treatment from another. (*Diseases* 1 22)

And thus,

> Medicine cannot be learned quickly because it is impossible to create any established principle in it, the way that a person who learns writing according to the single system people teach understands everything; for all who understand writing in the same way do so because the same symbol does not sometimes become opposite, but is always steadfastly the same and not subject to chance. Medicine, on the other hand, does not do the same thing at one moment and the next, and it does opposite things to the same person, and sometimes even things that are contradictory to one another. (*Places in Man* 41*;* cf. 42-46)

> There is no demonstrated starting point of healing, which truly is the starting point of the whole art (*techne*), nor any second point, nor any middle, or end. But rather we begin in it sometimes by speaking, at other times by acting, and we end in like manner; nor, when we begin by speaking, do we begin with the same words, not even if we are speaking about the same thing, nor do we end with the same words. In the same way, when we begin by acting, we do not begin with the same actions, nor do we end with the same ones. (*Diseases 1 9;* see chapters 1-10 in general)

But in spite of this complexity, or for that matter medicine's limited practical effectiveness—which was well appreciated—the enterprise is not to be abandoned as impossible, only accepted as being a difficult one. The clinical judgment that each practitioner must learn consists in appreciating both the value and the limits of rational thought in practice, and in knowing how to be guided by the individual patient's responses, even to the point of apparent theoretical nonsense, e.g.,

> If the (sc. hot) disease does not slacken when treated with cold compresses, switch over and use the leather skin to warm. (*Diseases* 2 16)

> . . . the principle would be established that sometimes conditions can be treated by things opposite to those from which they arose, and sometimes by things like to those from which they arose. (*Places in Man* 42)

From this methodological insecurity in practice there could not but follow a degree of professional insecurity. The physician was constantly in the position of applying an art whose results were open to more than one interpretation, e.g.,

> Generally speaking, people blame the physician, in diseases and wounds, even for the evils that follow of necessity from other evils, when these occur, not recognizing the constraint that makes such things happen. If he attends a patient with a fever or a wound, and fails at first to help him by his treatment, but on the next day the patient is worse, people blame the physician; but if he does help the patient, people do not praise him in due proportion, for they hold the patient's improvement to have been a matter of course. (*Diseases* 18)

In this difficult situation, writers sought to clarify the goals and responsibilities of the clinical intervention,

> . . . with these (sc. acute diseases) let nothing bad be added by the person treating —rather let the evils resulting from the diseases themselves suffice—but only whatever good he is capable of. If, when the physician treats correctly, the patient is overcome by the magnitude of his disease, this is not the physician's fault; but if, when the physician treats either incorrectly or out of ignorance, the patient is overcome, it is. (*Affections* 13)

and to define its parameters,

> As to diseases, make a habit of two things—to help, or at least to do no harm. The art has three factors, the disease, the patient, the physician: the physician is the servant of the art; the patient must work with the physician in combatting the disease. (*Epidemics* 1, 11)

If the medicine that emerges from this account seems, in spite of its obvious strengths, to be riven with contradictions between science and art, between theory and empiricism, between confidence and doubt, between naïveté and profundity, then it can rightfully take its place among its peer disciplines in classical Greek culture. This was an age when the ambiguity and ambivalence of human life in all its aspects were at the center of attention. On the one hand, "Man is the measure of all things, of the things that are, that they are, of the things that are not, that they are not" (Protagoras, Fragment 1). On the other, "There are many *deina* (marvellous, powerful, clever, dangerous, terrible) things in the world, but nothing is more *deinon* than man" (Sophocles, *Antigone* 332-333).

Hippocratic medicine, classical medicine, in striving to face openly the essential challenges that lie at the heart of the healing endeavor, presented all succeeding ages with a set of questions and potential answers that could never again go unasked or unfaced. When Thomas Sydenham, or René Laennec, or William Osler turn back to these writings in formulating their methods and seeking their models, they are not paying lip-service to a superceded historical stage in the development of their art. They are seeking help from an age which in some ways saw with a mental clarity never again achieved in the West, probed with an intellectual fortitude lost to its heirs. It is for this reason that they, and we, go back to Hippocrates.

Instead of a Bibliography

Greek and Latin editions accompanied by facing English translations of most ancient texts are available in the Loeb Classical Library published by Harvard University Press, Cambridge, Massachusetts. However, because many of these translations go back to the beginning of the present century and are in verse, they often fail to meet the requirements of the contemporary reader, who is better served by the less extensive but more modern series of translations published by Penguin Classics.

References to classical texts are generally standard in modern editions and translations, referring either to author, title, "book" and verse in poetry (e.g. Homer, *Iliad,* book 11, verse 514), and author, title, "book" and chapter in prose writers (e.g. Hippocrates, *Diseases of Women,* book 1, chapter 62), or to author, title, page and section in certain standard editions (e.g. Plato, *Protagoras,* page 311, section b, in the Stephanus edition of 1578, whose page and section numbers are indicated in the margins of all modern Plato editions).

In the two series mentioned in the first paragraph above, the ancient medical writers are not well represented, a situation which is being remedied to a degree by the addition of new volumes. The eight *Hippocrates* volumes in the Loeb series now contain over two thirds of the Hippocratic Collection, arranged more or less at random. For a general overview of the individual Hippocratic treatises and the medicine they represent, I refer the reader to Jacques Jouanna, *Hippocrates,* Baltimore, 1999, or more briefly, Paul Potter, *A Short Handbook of Hippocratic Medicine,* Quebec, 1988.

Health Care in the Next Millennium*

John David Stobo

John D. Stobo received his B.A. from Dartmouth College and his M.D. from the State University of New York at Buffalo. He completed an internship and assistant residency and served as chief medical resident on the Osler Medical Service of the Johns Hopkins Hospital in Baltimore.

After serving on the faculties of the Mayo Clinic and the Howard Hughes Medical Institute at the University of California, San Francisco, Dr. Stobo returned to Baltimore in 1985. A specialist in rheumatology and immunology, he served as the William Osler Professor of Medicine and director of the Department of Medicine at the Johns Hopkins University School of Medicine. He also served as physician-in-chief of the Johns Hopkins Hospital. Shortly thereafter, Dr. Stobo was chosen to lead the new Johns Hopkins Health Care LLC, which was charged with developing an integrated delivery system on behalf of Johns Hopkins Medicine. He then was also named vice dean for research and technology for the Johns Hopkins University School of Medicine.

In 1997, Dr. Stobo was named president of the University of Texas Medical Branch at Galveston, Texas' oldest health sciences university. He has been instrumental in bringing diverse areas of the university together to define UTMB's core values and shape its future as a leading center for health sciences education, medical research, and patient care.

Dr. Stobo is a member of the Institute of Medicine-National Academy of Sciences, and has chaired its board on health sciences policy. He is the past president of the American College of Rheuma-

*Delivered 5 May 1999 at the Twenty-ninth Annual Meeting of the American Osler Society, Montreal, Canada.

tology, past president of the Association of Professors of Medicine, and past chairman of the American Board of Internal Medicine. In 1996, he received a mastership from the American College of Physicians for his distinguished contributions to internal medicine.
Dr. Stobo and his wife, Mary Ann, have three children—John, Robert, and Heather—and three grandchildren.

It is an honor to present the John P. McGovern lecture at this, the 1999 American Osler Society annual meeting, and to be before this distinguished group.

Shortly after arriving in Galveston approximately eighteen months ago, I had the pleasure of meeting Jack McGovern. I soon learned that we share more than a first name. We share a commitment to the Oslerian principles of professionalism and, more importantly, a concern that these principles are under assault in a rapidly changing health care environment. Mention of medicine as a business, health care as a commodity, physician unions, and patients as covered lives gives credence to that concern. This concern serves as the impetus for my presentation to you: Health Care in the Next Millennium. What should the health care environment look like in the twenty-first century in order to preserve the principles of professionalism? What needs to be done to assure society that, as health professionals, we are acting in their—and not our—best interests? In other words, I would like to present my thoughts about changes that need to occur in the behavior of health professionals to reaffirm their commitment to serving the health needs of society.

To those of you who are waiting to hear specific prognostications on what reimbursement methodologies will be present in the future, whether or not everyone will carry their medical record on a smart card, or whether or not we will have a genetic profile of disease susceptibility determined at birth, I am sorry to say you will be disappointed. I am not going to talk about such specific changes. Instead, I will present general concepts to frame a health care environment in which the concepts of professionalism can flourish.

Before discussing the future, it is necessary to talk about the past: where medicine has come from. Indeed, American medicine has come a long way in the past hundred years.

At the turn of the last century, medicine in the United States hardly was struggling as a profession. The Flexner Report of 1910 pointed out that there were too many medical schools training too many physicians who were ill equipped to deal not only with the afflictions of society, but also to exemplify the tenets of professionalism.[1] The Flexner Report stated, "The medical profession has become diluted with practitioners of low ideals and professional honor." The report called on medical leadership to restore the principles of professionalism when it stated, "Those who represent the higher ideals of the medical profession must take a stand for that form of education calculated to advance the true interests of society and to better the ideals of medicine itself."

Fortunately, there was leadership in American medicine—William Osler being most prominent—which did reset the moral compass for medicine. The last hundred years have been characterized, until most recently, by advances that have enhanced the professional status of medicine. But, as I mentioned, now, as we approach the next century, the professional status of medicine faces significant challenges analogous to the situation that confronted medicine as it entered into this century.

What about the future? What should occur in the health care environment to preserve medicine's professional status?

The new health care environment should be framed by three concepts: community, collaboration, and curriculum—alliteration to frame a community-centric, cooperative health care system addressing health care needs and educating health profession students for tomorrow's medicine.

Community

The first concept to shape the new health care environment is community. In discussing the challenges faced by academic health centers and health sciences universities in the United States, I believe that only those entities that are viewed as adding value to the health of the communities they serve will indeed be successful in the future. In order to survive in the twenty-first century, health sciences universities will require public support. They will not get this support unless the geographic community they serve views them as adding value to the health of that community. Health sciences universities must be viewed as a community resource. Indeed, in the future, all health-related activities must move from egocentric entities to a community-centric coalition.[2] They must ask what is best for the community, not what is best for the individual entity. I believe that health sciences universities should be leaders in promulgating this community-centric orientation and organizing these community-centric coalitions.

This concept has several important implications. The coalition must have a governance structure that allows it to function as a community cooperative, with enlightened, dedicated community citizens making decisions as stewards of the health of the community. The bottom line will be the measured health status of the community and not the balance sheet of the hospital or other health-related entity. Chief executive officers, presidents, and other executive leaders will be judged by their ability to enhance the health status of the community and not by the profits and losses in their individual health care enterprise. The question will be what is ethical, not what is profitable. The individual health-related enterprises and the aggregate coalition must be viewed as being advocates for the unmet health needs of the community.

In the United States, there are some examples presently of health-related entities that are community-centric, and do have the governance structure of a community cooperative. For example, there is a group of approximately six hundred community clinics scattered throughout the country that are committed to addressing the unmet health needs of the community. They receive some support from the federal government. These federally qualified health centers are mandated to have at least 51 percent of their board made up of directors who utilize their services. I have worked with several federally qualified health centers and witnessed their community commitment. I have participated in their governance structure and seen the enormous benefit this structure brings to the center's ability to address community heath needs.

I submit that such a community cooperative governance structure, in the future, will be important for the oversight of health sciences universities. Rather than a board of directors or trustees, consisting of intelligent, well-meaning, and successful individuals who are selected predominantly because of their wealth and influence, the governance structure will change to consist of equally capable, local, community citizens. Only in this way will health sciences universities be seen as truly reaching out to address community health needs.

In this world of community-centric health care, there will be a painful clash of cultures and values as health-related institutions and their community boards make decisions about how to best allocate resources to ensure the greatest health care benefit to the largest number of individuals. They must move painfully from the traditional ways of making decisions based on wanting everything for each individual patient, to a paradigm in which decisions are based on how to use the available resources to provide the greatest good to the most people. The community rather than a single individual will become the "patient." A community-centric health care system will understand that advancing the health status of the community involves more than traditional health professionals and traditional delivery sites.[2] Preventive and health maintenance strategies and changes in lifestyle to advance health status cannot occur without the participation of a variety of health professionals and advanced-degree caregivers. While physicians play an important role in the health care delivery system, they will be part of a team including nurses, midwives, allied health professionals, public health officials, educators, and others.

The community-centric health care system will utilize existing community resources and facilities instead of requiring more and building new ones. The system will realize that a church or school can be a primary care clinic or screening site.[2]

Collaboration

In order for the community-centric health care system to work, it must embrace a second concept: collaboration. The health care environment must move from the present paradigm of competition to the new paradigm of collaboration. If health care is going to be community-centric, then all health providers, health facilities and agencies in the geographic community must come together in a coalition to take what is a fragmented, duplicative, inefficient, wasteful and expensive health care system, and transform it into a coordinated, efficient and cost-effective system to address community health needs.

Included in this coalition will be traditional health care providers as well as other disciplines and agencies that can have an impact on health needs but heretofore have not been part of the traditional health care mainstream. This includes schools, churches, transportation agencies, housing authorities, social services, and others.[2] Hospitals, which previously, through the paradigm of competition, have added costs to health care by replicating facilities and services, will come together to rationalize these same facilities and services in the context of what is best for the community, not what is best for the bottom line. In my opinion, there is no room for investor-owned health care providers or payors in such an environment. Fiduciary responsibility of the community-centric health system is to the health status of the community, not the financial betterment of shareholders. The community will not allow 10 to 15 cents of each health care dollar to be sent to Wall Street, when it can be best used locally to address health needs.

In selected areas of the United States there has already been some movement toward this new paradigm of cooperation instead of competition. This is being driven not only by the rising cost of health care and the realization that it is no longer financially possible to replicate costly facilities, technology and services, but also by the rapid increase in the United States of people who do not have health insurance—private or public—and cannot afford to pay for their care. Let me explain.

In the United States, beginning in the mid-1980s, there began an erosion in employer-based health insurance driven by yearly, near double-digit increases in health care costs. As health care costs and the costs of premiums increased, employers found it increasingly difficult to cover the cost of health insurance. They either stopped providing health insurance as an employee benefit or passed these costs on to employees. Employees, in turn, were not able to absorb these costs and stopped carrying health insurance. The result is that presently 15 percent of the U.S. population under the age of sixty-five—roughly 46 million Americans—cannot access the health care they need simply and solely because they lack heath insurance and cannot afford to pay for their care.[3] Even if they do get access to health care through emergency rooms and free clinics, it is fragmented, uncoordinated, and lacks emphasis on heath maintenance and prevention. Today, the number of uninsured in the United States is increasing by 1.5 million individuals each year.

The traditional health safety nets in the United States, particularly health sciences universities and their teaching hospitals, which provide 40 percent of the unsponsored care in the nation, are unable to accommodate the increasing number of uninsured.[4] This challenge of providing free care to the uninsured is therefore spilling over to health care entities that previously have not seen this as their problem. This situation is now having a negative financial impact on these entities, as well as the entities and agencies that traditionally have provided unsponsored care. Health-related facilities in specific geographical communities are now realizing that only by coming together in a cooperative coalition of health care providers and addressing the health needs of everybody in the community will they be able to weather the financial challenges of rising health care costs and the increasing number of uninsured. Let me provide a couple of examples.

Recently, I met with an executive of an investor-owned hospital in Texas. This executive related that there had been recent discussions with the executive leadership of a city-owned hospital that has historically served as a medical safety net for the community's unsponsored patients. The topic of the discussion was how both entities could work together to address the health needs of the community, including the uninsured. To me, this seemed to be an unlikely partnership, and when I asked why these discussions were taking place, the response was, "Because the numbers don't make sense anymore." In other words, because the balance sheets of both hospitals were suffering, leaders of both institutions realized that the survival of each required working together to address the financial concerns and the issue of providing health care to unsponsored patients. I predict this partnership, driven initially by financial motives, will be sustained by other, more altruistic ones.

A second example of a community-centric cooperative health system addressing unmet community health needs is a model system in the county of Hillsborough, Florida. In 1992, a coalition of providers in Hillsborough—consisting of five hospitals, one university medical association, two federally qualified health clinics, and a panoply of community providers and community services—came together to develop a health plan to provide health care to the uninsured of the county.[5] They started with a budget of $48 million (raised initially from an increase in the sales tax of a half cent). The plan initially provided health care to 28,000 uninsured. Five years later the plan had increased its enrollment to 50,000, with an increase of only $6 million in expenses. In five years, the plan had decreased the per-enrollee cost of delivering health care from $600 to $202 per month, decreased the number of admissions per 1000 enrollees from 134 to 12, decreased emergency room costs by $10 million, and had financial reserves of $156 million. Because the coalition was so successful financially, the needed sales tax was decreased from half to a quarter of a cent. Most importantly, the health status of the uninsured population, which initially had been significantly worse than that of the general population, was indistinguishable at the end of the five years from the health status of the general population.

This is a remarkable example of how a community of previously competitive health professionals and entities came together in a community-centric collaboration to address the problem of unsponsored care. In doing so, they decreased costs and improved the health of the community they served. I predict that soon the Hillsborough plan will need no additional tax subsidy. Instead, by controlling costs through appropriate utilization of health services and by increasing the health status of the community, they will be able to function using existing financial resources. Herein lies another important point. The environment of community-centric, collaborative health care, which will characterize the future, will result in a slowing of the yearly increases in health care costs.

Curriculum

The third concept framing the environment for the future is represented by the term curriculum. In order to meet the health needs of the community, the way we educate future generations of health professionals must change. In order to support a community-centric, cooperative health care environment, the curriculum should include topics that range from how to work as part of a cooperative venture to how to effectively address health needs of the community.[6] Topics related to teamwork, information management, continuous quality improvement, behavioral modification, health maintenance, prevention, efficient utilization of resources to address health needs of populations, ethics, spirituality in medicine, palliative care, end of life care—which are all making their way into traditional curricula for health professionals—will become core components of education in the health professions. Much of what is now termed alternative or complementary medicine will be demonstrated to contribute to a healing environment and included in the mainstream of therapeutics. The operative for determining how to approach a health issue will move from *do it right* to *do the right thing*. Outcomes, quality and what is best for the greater community will become benchmarks for success.

In addition to changing the curriculum used to educate health professionals for tomorrow's world, the way they are educated will change. Approaches that educate students as individual health professionals will not prepare them for the cooperative approach to health care. Classrooms of the twenty-first century will be virtual classrooms, educating diverse health professions students as a team, so that they can learn from each other as they come to understand that what the team contributes to the health of the community far exceeds the sum of what each contributes individually.

If there is to be a centennial repeat of the Flexner Report, it should examine how health professionals and entities, including health sciences universities, have come together to address the health needs of their communities. It should point to models, including health sciences universities that have developed model curricula and methods for educating teams of individuals to address health needs. Hopefully, the next Flexner Report will describe not only model experiments, but showcase health sciences universities that have led the formation of community-centric coalitions to better the health status of the community.

I began this presentation by commenting on how far American medicine has come in this century. As we now turn from this into the next century, there are certain similarities between the environment now, and that which existed as medicine transitioned from the nineteenth to the twentieth century. Medicine in the United States, now as then, is in turmoil. Like then, we seem to be in a transition of chaos and crisis. In the last transition, Flexner pointed the way by showcasing institutions in the United States that represented examples of what medical education, research, and clinical care should look like. The centennial Flexner Report should focus on communities and health sciences universities that have moved from a position of self-interest and competition, to one in which what matters most are the interests and well-being of the community. This Flexner Report will be the blueprint for our ability to sustain the principles of professionalism. Those we serve will indeed understand that we as health professionals are acting in their best interests.

I want to thank you for the privilege of coming before you and I especially want to thank Jack McGovern, not only for his generous support of American medicine but also for reminding us that, in the words of Osler, "We are in this profession as a calling, not as a business; as a calling which extracts from us at every turn self-sacrifice, devotion, love and tenderness to our fellow man. We must work in the missionary spirit with a breath of charity that raises us far above the petty jealousies in life."[7]

References

1. Flexner, A. *Medical Education in the United States and Canada. A Report to the Carnegie Foundation for the Advancement of Teaching*. Boston, Merrymount Press, 1910.
2. Bezold, C. and Mayer, E. Future Care: *Responding to the Demand for Change*. New York, Faulkner & Gray, 1996.
3. Kuttner, R. The American health care system. Health insurance coverage. *N Engl J Med* 340: 163-168, 1999.
4. Igglehart, J.K. The American health care system. Expenditures. *N Engl J Med* 340: 70-76, 1999.
5. Cole, M., and Johnson, C. *Hillsborough HealthCare Annual Report*, February, 1998.
6. O'Neil, E.H., and the Pew Health Professions Commission. San Francisco, Pew Health Professions Commission. December, 1998.
7. Holman, E. Osler and Halsted, a Contrast in Personalities. In: *Humanism in Medicine*, McGovern, J.P. and Burns, C.R. (Eds.), Springfield, IL, Charles C. Thomas, 1973, pp. 21-29.

"Writ Large": Medical History, Medical Anthropolgy, and Medicine and Literature*

Gert Henry Brieger

Gert H. Brieger, is Distinguished Service Professor, Department of the History of Medicine, The Johns Hopkins University School of Medicine. Previously he served as the William H. Welch Professor and Chairman of the Department. He received his M.D. in 1957 at UCLA; M.P.H in 1962 at Harvard University School of Public Health, and Ph.D in 1968 at the Johns Hopkins University. After several years of family practice, Dr. Brieger turned to medical history which he has taught at Duke, the University of California, San Francisco, and at the Johns Hopkins University.

Dr. Brieger's interests are in the history of American medicine and public health, the history of surgery, and the history of medical education. He edited *Medical America in the Nineteenth Century* (1972), and *Theory and Practice in American Medicine . . .* (1976). Other works include *Human Experimentation: History* (1978) and *Mitral Valve Stenosis: A Case Study in the History of Surgery* (1984). With A. McGhee Harvey, S.H. Abrams and Victor A. McKusick, he authored *A Model of Its Kind, A Centennial History of Johns Hopkins Medicine*, 2 Vols. (1993). Since 1990, Dr. Brieger has served as editor of the *Bulletin of the History of Medicine.* Currently, he is completing a book on the history of premedical education in America. He is past president of the American Association for the History of Medicine.

*Delivered 17 May 2000 at the Thirtieth Annual Meeting of the American Osler Society, Bethesda, Maryland.

In this presentation, I want to discuss the writing of medical history. That this was also an important preoccupation for William Osler makes my subject even more appropriate. While Osler's history was in a different style from ours, he was not afraid of new ideas or new ways of seeing old things.

As Michael Bliss has noted in his wonderful new biography of Osler,[1] much of Osler's historical work led him to the present concerns of his time. And so, too, is this true for many of us. Osler himself said, in his lectures at Yale that became *The Evolution of Modern Medicine,* "To understand the old writers one must see as they saw, feel as they felt, believe as they believed—and this is hard, indeed impossible."[2] He also said that while we have need for literary history, we have no use for literary criticism. But were he here today to observe how his beloved history of medicine has expanded in so many ways, I believe he too would have seen the potential of this newer history of medicine, one writ large, or at least larger than in his day.

My purpose in this McGovern Lecture is not to probe William Osler's historiographical style, nor is it to defend the various new ways of seeing or writing the history of medicine. I would merely like to draw your attention to some interesting developments in our neighboring fields of inquiry, particularly the relatively new ones of medicine and literature, and medical anthropology. But before doing so, let me say just a word about the use of the English language.

Language and its uses is a connecting theme among the many books I will mention or discuss. Language is also an important theme in Osler's work, and he was generally meticulous in its use. After a decade in an editor's chair, I admit that I have become less patient with the careless use of words and with jargon. I do realize that language changes and evolves, but I find it particularly distressing when our colleagues who are professors of English tell us they are essentializing, problematizing, privileging, and foregrounding. Lord knows, medicine has been known to hide behind its own jargon in order to maintain distance or mystique, and I do not like that any better. Why not say it clearly, to borrow from the title of a little book by Lester King?[3]

The origin of this lecture is in two very long essay reviews I have been writing for the *Bulletin of the History of Medicine,* each attempting to capture for our readers the richness of these two burgeoning tangential fields—medicine and anthropology, and medicine and literature. Indeed, as we shall see, it is not always a simple task to assign a book to one or the other group. What both groups of authors have in common is that they believe that their approach to understanding the human condition will enrich the work of physicians and historians. The anthropologist and the literary critic, both with and without their jargon, have become an important part of the intellectual scene of these last two decades, and so surely it behooves those of us trying to make sense of medicine's past and present to take their work into account. In the good Galenic sense of eclecticism we need to see what these authors and their books have to offer us, to take what is of use, and to reject, at least for now, what we deem not useful. Notice that I did not say "useless," for one of the lessons of interdisciplinary studies might well be to dismiss the notion of dismissiveness; when it comes to broadening our understanding of the roles and meanings of illness in our lives.

Highlighting the work of our colleagues in medical anthropology should not seem novel to the readers of the *Bulletin.* We are, after all, the inheritors of a rich tradition emphasized in the work of Henry E. Sigerist, our founding editor. And it was he who published here many of the papers on primitive medicine by Erwin Ackerknecht.

In more recent times, however, it has been the social historians who have "plundered the works of French and British anthropologists . . ." in the words of the historian Michael MacDonald.[4] Despite the potential usefulness of the anthropological perspective for the history of science and medicine, MacDonald had to admit, in 1983, that the promise was yet greater than the practice, for, "Historians of science and medicine have not shown much interest in these clamorous raids into alien territory."[5] A decade and a half later, new work in the history of international health (or what used to be called tropical medicine) emphasizes cultural strands, but it is probably still fair to say that our anthropological colleagues have a better appreciation for what we have written in the history of medicine than we have of their work. Hence one justification for some discussion of a group of recent books on medical anthropology. The choice of examples is mostly driven by what has been sent to the *Bulletin* for review, but is representative of a vibrant field. All of the books included in my discussion clearly demonstrate MacDonald's point that these works "should interest historians because they offer fresh discussions of the ways in which knowledge is organized and expressed in speech and action."[6]

Medical anthropology, a term first used in the early 1960s, has a much longer history. Rudolf Virchow and Paul Broca in the mid-nineteenth century were active in physical anthropology. Earlier in this century, W.H.R. Rivers and Erwin Ackerknecht were also physicians who turned to social anthropology. Despite the ensuing expansion of medical anthropology, in scope of work and numbers of workers, Byron Good recalls that "in the 1960s, it was something of an embarrassment to be identified as a medical anthropologist. Medical anthropology was largely a practice discipline in those days . . . committed to putting anthropology at the service of improving the public health of societies in the third world."[7]

In their 1978 book about medical anthropology, George Foster and Barbara Anderson described four roots of the contemporary field of medical anthropology: the interests of physical anthropologists in evolution, comparative anatomy, and racial types; ethnographic interest in witchcraft and primitive medicine; the culture and personality movement of the 1930s; and the international public health movement after World War II.[8] It is the last of these that has had a particularly strong influence on our work in the history of medicine. I should also point out that both anthropologists and historians have addressed the relationship of these two disciplines, for example, the medical anthropologists John and Jean Comaroff, in their book *Ethnography and the Historical Imagination.*[9]

Much has been written in the last two or three decades about the rich relation of medicine and literature. Their common bonds will become even more evident as we proceed. Since both medicine and literature are humanistic arts whose object is to study and to understand the human condition, it hardly needs to be said that both the stories of our patients as well as those we read in novels or stories serve to enhance our perceptive skills and to broaden and enrich our understanding of human nature.

Nearly twenty years ago, I wrote, "Good literature can contribute greatly to the effectiveness of those in the health professions, since literature, like their own work, is concerned with human activity and human values. One of the essentials of any education is that it should help us to go beyond or to transcend our own limited experiences and make us sensitive to the world of others. History and literature can help us to do this. . . . Literature is as good a source for the study of life histories as any clinic, for in good literature we not only see the bare facts of illness, but have in addition the writer's interpretation of their meaning for the patient. It is the interpretive skill that makes up a good part of the art of medicine as it does literature."[10] Or, as Martha Nussbaum has said, "all living is interpreting."[11] In the nearly two decades since my essay appeared, the importance of the humanities in medicine has grown. A continuing discussion of the profession's core values and consideration of our recent as well as our more distant history have increased because of the rapidly changing world of medical practice and medical science. Decisions, both large and small, require constant attention to both social and biological contexts. To the latter, we devote much of our precious years of collegiate and medical education. Our colleagues in the humanities and the social sciences have done much to enrich our understanding of the social context of health and disease, thereby helping us to help our patients to cope with illness. Good literature, then, as Dean Silva of Martin Arrowsmith's medical school put it, will help us to become "passionate on behalf of mankind."[12]

Medicine, we might argue, deals with "facts," while literature is usually fiction— or, as the Canadian novelist Margaret Atwood has more colorfully said it, writers of fiction "concoct whoppers, which they hope they can induce the public to swallow whole."[13] Yet the writer of fiction and the writer of medical case histories, the physician, must both learn to exercise their skills of interpretation. For the writer, these skills lead to successful stories. For the physician much more than good reviews or large sales rides on the clinical interpretation. For the patient what is at stake is a correct diagnosis on which subsequent treatment is usually based.

There are some themes that are common to many of these new books about health and illness in present and past cultures. Some of the themes I want to discuss include interdisciplinarity; narrative, language, and discourse; women's health; the body; pain and suffering; medical education; and evolutionary theory. It is important to note that these are the province of historians, and are not unique to medical anthropologists or those who write about medicine and literature. Gina Morantz-Sanchez, for instance, discusses virtually all of them in her recent book about Dr. Mary Dixon Jones and the evolution of gynecological surgery.[14]

Interdisciplinarity

My first theme is interdisciplinarity, or boundary crossing. This was discussed by Michel Foucault in his many works and found explicit expression in the anthropologist Clifford Geertz's widely cited essay of 1980, "Blurred Genres: The Reconfiguration of Social Thought."[15]

"In recent years," Geertz wrote, "there has been an enormous amount of genre mixing in social science as in intellectual life generally, and such blurring is continuing apace." This was not merely a redrawing of the cultural map, Geertz maintained, but, "something is happening to the way we think about the way we think."

One result of this "genre mixing" is the appearance of books spanning several fields. *Morality and Health,* for example, is a series of essays by medical historians, sociologists, and anthropologists.[16] Edited by Allan Brandt and Paul Rozin, the book emerged from a conference of an interdisciplinary network sponsored by the MacArthur Foundation to study the behavioral, social, and cultural determinants of health and disease. Clearly, no single discipline is adequate to account for such complexities.

Science in the late twentieth century is generally accorded a distinctive niche in our intellectual ecosystem, according to Thomas Gieryn.[17] Yet boundary disputes continue to occur, as in the heated discussions raised by creationism or alternative medicine. Boundary maintenance becomes a turf battle when a profession (or any occupational group) wishes to expand its authority into areas claimed by other groups, when it tries to maintain a monopoly of its work so that outsiders are called amateurs, or when it wishes to exempt its members from the responsibility for the consequences of their work by putting blame for mishaps or failure on scapegoats from the outside.

Narrative

A second pervasive theme in the history of medicine writ large is its emphasis upon the use of language, on discourse and narrative. Historians of all kinds, as well as sociologists and anthropologists, have for some years been discussing a "linguistic turn" in their work. This implies an interest not only in what is said or written, but in what context and with what interpretive framework.

We are a narrative species, Kathryn Hunter reminds us.[18] We constantly tell stories, listen to them, and watch them. Our human experiences, including those we tell to our doctors, are the stuff of narrative. Narrative, then, is the way we make sense of the world. As the clinical narrative tells us much about the patient's illness, so the way we tell our history of medical ideas and practices indicates a great deal about how we perceive ourselves as an occupational group, as a profession, as healers.

Julia Epstein's *Altered Conditions: Disease, Medicine, and Storytelling*[19] is an especially apt illustration of how the literary scholar approaches the history of medicine. Here a professor of comparative literature writes a series of well-crafted and well-researched essays on the cultural history of medicine. Taking her title from the mid-nineteenth century work of Rudolf Virchow, Epstein has taken on the question of how western cultures have produced and used medical narratives about the body within the medical domain. She contends that explanatory stories about the body are used to contain people in safe and recognized boundaries of social norms. She discusses definitions of disease, the development of medical record-keeping, and the various styles of medical narratives. With each of her essays, she provides a very useful bibliographic discussion of what has been written about these subjects since the eighteenth century. Thus Epstein sketches the history of medical storytelling. Despite her own literary background—and in contrast to books like Miriam Bailin's *The Sickroom in Victorian Fiction*,[20] and Athena Vrettos's *Somatic Fictions*[21]—she makes greater use of nonfiction than fictional works. It is Epstein's critical reading that I want to emphasize here. While she does not break new historical ground in her book (which includes essays on hermaphroditism, maternal impressions and birth malformations, and AIDS), her provocative examples make this an important and useful work.

A particularly telling example of the importance of close reading comes in her first chapter, where she is concerned with defining disease. Here Epstein cites an opening sentence of a 1991 article, in the *Archives of Physical Medicine and Rehabilitation,* about the AIDS epidemic, to show how important careful writing and careful reading may be: "In only a decade the acquired immune deficiency syndrome (AIDS) has evolved from a novel immune deficiency disorder of unknown etiology in homosexual men to an infectious disease of pandemic proportions that has challenged the basic fabric of society."[22] An unremarkable sentence, one we encounter often, we might say. Yet Epstein calls to our attention several aspects of this sentence that reveal much about how we perceive this disease. For example, when AIDS strikes gay men, it is a disorder, but when it affects everybody else it becomes an infectious disease caused by a pathogen in the blood. What is of even greater significance is that, probably unwittingly, the author implies that homosexual men do not participate in the basic fabric of society. Much discourse about women, minorities, and many "others" in our culture could doubtless be analyzed in a similar way. Thus it is a lesson we may learn from our literary colleagues: that language matters; that while we generally consider ourselves to be humane, to have only the best of intentions, our discourse often belies something else.

There is, of course, another possible reading of the sentence in question, as one constructed mainly for stylistic purpose. Epstein's premise in her book is that "narrative desire–the human drive to tell stories—underlies the ways we construct the so-called normal and the aberrant, and the ways we explain disjunctions between the two."[23]

As another example of the importance of narrative, Epstein traces the history of the medical record, showing how the professional discourse of medicine has evolved. As my colleague Mary Fissell has noted, early in the eighteenth century the words of doctors and their patients were one. "But over the course of the century, this symmetry fades. Doctors begin to sound like doctors, and patients' voices disappear."[24] It is through the record of a case that the patient is converted to a medical problem, to which the full powers of the new diagnostic and therapeutic medicine can then be brought into play. Modern case records date from the eighteenth century. They were developed for a variety of reasons and purposes— for teaching, administrative, financial, legal, and statistical compilations.

Narrative is an implicit or explicit theme in virtually all of our books. Some, such as Arthur Frank's *The Wounded Storyteller,*[25] describe narratives as central to the doctor-patient encounter. The sick patient, Frank tells us, undergoes a narrative surrender when the doctor's version of the illness story takes over from the patient's version. It is this surrender that is reversed in so-called postmodern illness when patients have once again taken command of their fate.

Frank describes three main narrative types of illness stories: the "restitution narrative" dominates the stories of most sick people who wish to be restored to health. The "chaos narrative" features an antithetical plot: the patient imagines that life will never get better. (Frank calls this a "narrative wreckage.") The third type of narrative in Frank's scheme is the "quest narrative," in which an attempt is made to hold chaos at bay. This type of narrative affords patients a distinctive voice and is the type of narrative found in most published illness narratives written by patients or their families.

These types of patient and family narratives are fully described and well analyzed by Anne Hawkins in her book *Reconstructing Illness: Studies in Pathography*.[26]

Women's Health

A thorough discussion of women and their illnesses in the nineteenth century appears in Diane Price Herndl's *Invalid Women: Figuring Feminine Illness in American Fiction and Culture, 1840-1940*.[27] Along with Elaine Showalter's

Hystories: Hysterical Epidemics and Modern Media[28] and Lilian R. Furst's *Between Doctors and Patients: The Changing Balance of Power*[29] Herndl's is the most explicitly medical history in its attempt to describe medical practices as they relate to half the population. Using both medical and literary sources, Herndl persuasively argues that female illness (whether sentimental, manipulative, or otherwise) is perceived in a male world as strongly negative. So strong have been male prejudices, she claims, that women have had "to prove they are not feigning illness before they can be taken seriously."

Herndl is correct, I believe, in pointing out that many of our society's current health problems-such as high infant mortality, poverty in its relationship to sickness, and care for the elderly—are all women's issues. She shows us the many varieties of the representation of illness, as attempts to seek attention or power, as real or imagined. All may be found in the texts she analyzes for us.

In the mid-nineteenth century, Herndl claims, physicians gained access to the American household by means of the woman of the house. The texts she discusses include many novels; she also gives us sensitive readings of such contemporary tracts as Edward H. Dixon's *Woman and Her Diseases, from the Cradle to the Grave; Adapted Exclusively to Her Construction in the Physiology of Her System and All the Diseases of Her Critical Periods* (1847)[30] and *Sex in Education,* written in 1873 by Edward H. Clarke.[31] This book generated a vigorous feminist response, including a widely distributed essay by Dr. Mary Putnam Jacobi[32] and no less than four books published within a year. Male physicians did indeed have an economic interest in the illnesses of their women patients, but to claim that they deliberately kept them in an invalid state is no easy thing to prove—and Herndl is not successful, I believe.

Other notable books on the subject of women's health include Mary Wood's *The Writing on the Wall: Women's Autobiography and the Asylum,*[33] which, written by a professor of English, is as much a contribution to the history of the care of the mentally ill as it is to the imaginative use of literary works to elucidate that history. Lilian Furst, author of *Between Doctors and Patients,* devotes a section to five American novels about women physicians, all published within a decade, 1881-1891. Furst compares these novels with British counterparts (including a story by Arthur Conan Doyle), all published at about the same time. The American novels were William Dean Howells's, *Dr. Breen's Practice;*[34] *Dr. Zay,* by Elizabeth Stuart Phelps[35]; *A Country Doctor,* by Sarah Orne Jewett;[36] *The Bostonians,* [37] by Henry James; and Annie Nathan-Meyer's *Helen Brent, M.D* [38] I should add that Furst is not the first to write about these novels; Chester Burns and others have done so in the past.[39]

Furst elucidates the many parallel themes in these books about women physicians at the end of the nineteenth century. There was surprise at the very idea of a woman practicing medicine; doubts about propriety for a well-brought-up woman; the dilemma of marriage and a career; and a schism between the newer, scientific style of medicine and what Furst calls the "redemptive style." These novels about medical women, Furst claims, have a dual significance: they are the literary exposition of the vexed "woman question," and for medicine as a whole, they expose the conflict between the new, scientific medicine and the traditional practice—or what she refers to as the missionary to the bedside, the redemptive style of medical practice.

The Body

In a glowing introduction to Peter Logan's *Nerves and Narratives,* Roy Porter puts it succinctly: "One of the most exciting recent developments in the humanities has been the interaction between literary criticism and the history of medicine, mediated through studies of the body."[40] Or, as David Arnold so aptly put it in his study of the role medicine played in the colonization of India, "The history of medicine in European and North American societies over the past two hundred years has been a history of growing intervention and a quest for monopolistic rights over the body."[41]

Scholarly interest in studies of the body greatly increased in the last two to three decades. This interest reflects the influence of Michel Foucault, who showed us clearly that one route to power was through knowledge of the body. More recent interest in the body emerges in books on beauty by Naomi Wolf,[42] and in *The Body Project,* by historian Joan Brumberg, who traces the rich history of fads and fashions of the body of American girls and women.[43] Changing the body through the techniques of plastic surgery is the subject of books by Elizabeth Haiken[44] and Sander Gilman.[45] Gilman also wrote about *The Jew's Body,* in which plastic surgery of the nose plays a prominent part.[46] *Body Talk: Rhetoric, Technology, Reproduction,* by Mary M. Lay et al.,[47] combines the themes of language and body.

This rediscovery of the body as a subject of scholarly discourse is evident throughout virtually all of the books I am discussing. The body as a story or a text that can be read and interpreted as we do literary texts; the sick body; the well body; the gendered body; the narrative body; all make their appearance.[48,49] What has been particularly noteworthy in these last two decades has been the crossing of traditional boundaries of disciplines. We now find professors of English like Peter Logan[50] and Mary Poovey,[51] for instance, writing some of the most interesting commentary about Edwin Chadwick's famous sanitary report of 1842[52] as they describe the social and the political body.

Laura Otis, who turned from graduate work in the neurosciences to literary studies, became intrigued by physicians who not only wrote about their medical or scientific work but also turned to writing fiction. She discusses the work of Ramon y Cajal, S. Weir Mitchell, Arthur Conan Doyle, and Arthur Schnitzler. How did these writer-physicians handle such concepts as "identity" in comparison with scientists like Koch or Virchow, who stayed mainly with technical writing (though the latter was both an accomplished anthropologist and historian)? Otis's recent work, *Membranes: Metaphors of Invasion in Nineteenth-Century Literature, Science and Politics*[53] concerns borders of the cell state and the political state. As pathologists and bacteriologists defined and redefined the borders of individuals between 1830 and 1930, their governments were doing the same. That hundred-year period marked the spread of the Europeans beyond their borders to colonies in Africa and Asia. As Otis points out, the imperial powers marked the new territories and resources as "theirs," but the peoples and the diseases they encountered in these colonies were distinctly "not theirs." Thus as science was increasingly elaborating self and not-self, imperialism opened and expanded borders, and to some extent shifted traditional identities.

One of the metaphors Otis employs to good effect is that of the permeable membrane (hence her title). Immigration, on both sides of the Atlantic, for different reasons and from different sources, became a fierce political issue. The membranes were not quite so permeable when it came time to exclude colonials, or in the case of the United States, those coming from Europe.

Of the many possible bodily dichotomies, such as tall and short, fat and thin, old and young, or beautiful and ugly, none has more salience for medicine (and for society as a whole) than the able and disabled body. Thus disability studies among anthropologists, sociologists, and literary scholars have become increasingly prominent. While many books in both medical anthropology and literary theory touch on the body and its ailments, some are also devoted to disability.

Although race, gender, and class have come under increasing scrutiny in the last few decades, only recently has attention been focused on another isolating category, another way that we define difference: disability. As Robert Murphy, a professor of anthropology at Columbia, who was paralyzed for nearly fifteen years before his death in 1990, put it bluntly,

> The recently disabled paralytic faces the world with a changed body and an altered identity ? which even by itself would make his re-entry into society a delicate and chancy matter. But his future is made even more perilous by the way he is treated by the non-disabled, including some of his oldest friends and associates. . . . The greatest impediment to a person's taking full part in his society is not his physical flaws, but rather the issue of myths, fears, and misunderstanding that society attaches to them.[54]

Murphy and other writers point to the work of Erving Goffman, particularly his 1963 book, *Stigma: Notes on the Management of Spoiled Identity*,[55] as one of the intellectual stimuli. But the social and political consequences of the social activism of the 1960s also prepared the ground for the new field of disability studies.

Rosemary Thomson, a professor of English at Howard University, herself suffering from a physical disability, wants to bring disability studies beyond the social sciences and medicine, where they are well developed, to the humanities as well. Disability, she maintains, is too often discussed in exclusionary terms. In contrast, she perceives disability as a form of ethnicity. In her book *Extraordinary Bodies,* [56] she begins with a fascinating chapter on the role of freak shows in nineteenth-century and early twentieth-century American culture. She then examines several well-known literary texts, novels such as Harriet Beecher Stowe's *Uncle Tom's Cabin,*[57] Rebecca Harding Davis' *Life in the Iron Mills,*[58] and Elizabeth Stuart Phelps's *The Silent Partner.*[59] The freak shows were a form of entertainment, and they sensationalized disability. The sentimental fiction, on the other hand, validated it. The main purpose of these three mid-nineteenth century novels was to argue for a humanitarian social reform in major cultural and economic institutions of the time, such as slavery, the iron mill, and the textile industry. Each of the novels also featured a disabled woman as one of the characters. These disabled women do not prevail, as their "normal" sisters do. In these works, the authors hoped to move their readers from complacency to conviction. Thomson[56] also devotes a chapter to the discussion of disabled women in the more recent fiction of Ann Petry, Audre Lorde, and Toni Morrison.

Thus as Thomson, and some of our other authors show, the discourse of disability is but one of multiple narratives of identity, along with those of gender, race, ethnicity, privilege, and poverty.

Finally, in this genre of disability studies, we come to two sizable collections that are rich in case studies and interpretations. *The Body and Physical Difference: Discourses of Disability* was edited by David Mitchell and Sharon Snyder.[60] The editors and their fourteen contributors are mostly professors of English, although professors of German literature, ancient history, and the history of medicine (Martin Pernick) are also among the authors.

Two of the essays are especially noteworthy. David D. Yuan writes about a story of Oliver Wendell Holmes and the Palmer Leg as a prosthesis for wounded soldiers in the Civil War.[61] Other writers have traced the beginnings of rehabilitation medicine to the years right after World War I. Yuan here clearly demonstrates its Civil War roots. Caroline Molina's "Muteness and Mutilation, The Aesthetics of Disability in Jane Campion's *The Piano*"[62] is a sensitive reading of the film, which won three academy awards. The film highlighted some of the stereotypes associated with disability, particularly the relationship of muteness, physical deformity, and mental illness. A beautiful, erotic adventure of a woman who became suddenly speechless when her husband was killed, it shows us how the woman then expressed herself mainly through her piano and her daughter. Eventually she found love and regained her speech, and then had no more need of the piano that had been her link to the world of sound.

Disability and Culture, edited by Benedicte Ingstad and Susan R. Whyte,[63] is a collection of fourteen articles by anthropologists, almost all working in Scandinavian countries. These ethnographic studies were carried out in Africa, England, and Latin America, and they also discuss "historical changes in conception and practices related to disability." The excellent introduction by the editors and outstanding epilogue, "Disability between Discourse and Experience" by Professor Susan Whyte makes this volume central to our wider understanding of disability in the history of medicine.

Pain and Suffering

Pain, as several of our authors have pointed out, is one of the most frequent reasons for patients to seek medical help. It is not surprising, then, that pain is a theme in many of our books, especially those written by anthropologists. As David Morris has argued in his prize-winning book, *The Culture of Pain,* this phenomenon is always more than the organic model of nerves, the brain, and neurotransmitters.[64] What we need, he stresses, is to recover the voices of those who mainstream medicine has far too often left unheard, especially those with chronic pain.

To Aristotle pain was an emotion, like joy. Descartes saw it as a sensation, like heat or cold. Although doctors in all areas have been concerned with pain, never before in human history, Morris maintains, has pain fallen so completely into medical hands as it has in our time. We cannot simply suffer pain; we are compelled to make sense of it. And it is to medicine we turn for explanation as well as for help to alleviate it. But, as Morris points out, the uncomfortable truth is that doctors know far less about pain than their patients assume.

The social, political, and economic aspects of pain are usually subsumed under the related condition of suffering. As much as any of the books we are considering in these reviews, *Social Suffering,* edited by Arthur Kleinman, Veena Das, and Margaret Lock,[65] exemplifies the crossing of disciplinary boundaries. It would in any case seem difficult to draw any strict limits in a discussion of a subject as broad as suffering. The editors point out in their introduction that "social suffering results from what political, economic, and institutional power does to people." Legal, moral, religious, and health issues also usually occur simultaneously. "Trauma, pain, and disorder to which atrocity gives rise," they continue, "are health conditions; yet they are also political and cultural matters."[66]

Similarly, poverty is a major risk factor for ill health and death. Health, then, is a social indicator, especially in most of the world where biomedicine does not reign supreme. Far more important than technical medicine for most of the world's population are peace, prosperity, and plumbing.

The eighteen essays in this volume range from the Holocaust to Mao's

China, and to the suffering caused by AIDS in Haiti. These essays clearly demonstrate the importance of examining the relationship between language and pain and suffering. And much like the notion of permeable membranes, the authors describe the passage back and forth across the boundaries between bodies and social processes, between individual and social suffering, and the many possible relations of the body to misery and pain.

As Arthur and Joan Kleinman forcefully point out in their essay, when we look around at the world we can easily become "overwhelmed by the sheer number of atrocities. There is too much to see, and there appears to be too much to do anything about."[67] It is easy to see how moral exhaustion can set in. Yet we need to ask how victims of violence become patients with the social status such pathology then implies. And can we avoid distraction from spectacular violence abroad to focus on the misery we may see at home, if we but look around us to see it?

Medical Education

Another theme I want to discuss is the education of doctors. In one way or another, many of the books on literature and anthropology are concerned with bringing a greater understanding of health and illness to their readers. The anthropologist Cecil Helman's *Culture, Health, and Illness,*[68] and the many works of Arthur Kleinman,[65,69] both of whom are both medically and anthropologically qualified, speak to the doctor's need to understand what has happened to patients. Two other anthropologists, Robert Hahn,[70] and Howard Stein, [71] have spent years studying the role of doctors in present-day medical settings in this country. Hahn's ethnography of the day-to-day life and work of a general internist, [70] is informative for any reader who wants to experience a doctor's daily routine.

But it is the work of the husband and wife team of Byron Good and Mary Jo Good of Harvard Medical School's Department of Social Medicine that is especially informative. In chapters in both their respective books,[72,73] and in a jointly authored chapter in a collection,[74] the Goods provide us with an ethnography of how students learn medicine in Harvard's New Pathway. Their long descriptions of how students cope with new information, new language, and new responsibilities, make it clear that the Goods know as much about the Harvard medical education as anyone, with the possible exception of the students themselves (although Byron Good actually attended the first-year classes). Thus it seems strange indeed that their name is nowhere to be found in a recent "official" history of the New Pathway venture.[75]

In their jointly authored chapter, the Goods bring a new emphasis to the study of medical education, an anthropological perspective. In contrast to the older sociological literature, such as *The Student Physician*[76] or *Boys in White,*[77] which focus upon the socialization of students into a professional role, the Goods explore how medical knowledge is constructed during the learning process. They are less concerned with how students learn to play the role of doctor than with how they learn medical reasoning, how they come to know what they know.

The New Pathway at the Harvard Medical School began in 1984 with a group of twenty-four students, but soon expanded to include the entire class. The two perspectives of the New Pathway were an educational philosophy based upon the case method, and tutorial teaching and learning, and a vision of the physician of the twenty-first century as a continuing learner in a changing world of medical practice and information.

The students they observed and interviewed at length exhibited continuing concern with both competence and caring. The concern about becoming competent, "Will I know enough to help my patients effectively?" had been prevalent among medical students long before the advent of the New Pathway, but Good and Good evaluate it in finer detail than have previous studies of medical education. Competence, they note, has often been associated with the natural sciences, caring with the humanities.

They also discuss the common comparison of medical education with learning a foreign language. But they unearth a subtext: "Learning the language of medicine," they conclude, "consists not of learning new words for the common sense world, but the construction of a new world altogether."[78]

The humanities and the social sciences have contributed to the continuing dual discourse of competence and caring. And this leaves them in a somewhat precarious position. Good and Good conclude that anthropology in the medical schools has also played a critical role—as critic of the mechanistic approach of the biomedical sciences, of the social organization of medicine, and of the "nostalgic view of the human sciences as the providers of caring."[79]

While Byron focuses in his own book on the studies of the first year, Mary Jo pays more attention to the clinical years of medical education. Her book *American Medicine: The Quest for Competence*[73] is divided into three ethnographic studies that shed much light on contemporary medicine and how it is taught, learned, practiced, and perceived by both patients and their doctors.

The first and longest section of her book concerns rural practice in a coastal town in Northern California, and focuses especially on the relationship of family practitioners and obstetricians in an era of high malpractice insurance and real risk of legal encounters. It is in her second section, that Good describes how in their clinical years Harvard medical students learn to achieve competence. In the final section, she describes a project on the clinical narratives of patients with breast cancer.

This book will broaden the understanding of medical practice, medical politics, and medical education so necessary for historical work. By using competence as a core symbol, much as using response to disease outbreaks as a sampling device, Good can discuss issues such as authority, curriculum, and practice patterns in the evolution of medicine in America as we see it today. She describes three professional voices (which may be heard, for instance, in the debates about malpractice). The intraprofessional voice is used for dialogue with other members of the profession; an extraprofessional repertoire is used to mediate between the profession and the public; and a reflective repertoire is the language used by individual doctors or students to explore the experiences and meanings of competence and incompetence.[73]

Two other books concerned with teaching the humanities to medical students deserve special notice. The first is *Teaching Literature and Medicine.* Edited by Anne Hawkins and Marilyn McEntyre,[80] both professors of English who have taught medical students, it is a rich collection of experiences in a wide variety of course formats with many literary sources suitable for inclusion in such courses. This book, just published by the Modern Language Association, is not only a source of references, with ideas for teaching and model courses; it is also full of interpretations of literary works and insights into both medicine and human nature that surely will enrich both students and potential instructors alike.

From my own experience in teaching a course in medicine and literature, I urge other members of medical faculties who have a literary bent to do the same. This book of four hundred pages can serve as an invaluable guide. Books by Robert Coles,[81] Howard Brody,[82] and Kathryn Hunter [83] will likewise guide you.[84]

Medical students who were readers before they got caught up in the whirlwind of learning the biomedical sciences often wish they could continue to read novels and stories. An elective course gives them a structure in which to do it. William Osler was correct when he said, "literary criticism is not what we want."[85] I don't pretend that I can take a novel apart and put it together again as my literary colleagues can do so elegantly. Medical students, I have found, are eager to read and just as eager to talk about what they have read. How a book or story resonates with their lives, their concerns and needs, is what it is all about.

Culture, Health and Illness, by Dr. Cecil Helman,[68] is another excellent book for teaching medical students, social scientists, and humanists who want to learn about medicine. It first appeared in 1984; a second edition appeared in 1990; and a third in 1994. In the decade between the first and third editions the field of medical anthropology expanded greatly. As a result, both physicians and historians now take a more global view of health. At the same time, there has been a steady, growth of interest in medical anthropology among both social scientists and health professionals.

Of the many books I have chosen for review, three were written by physicians (Cecil Helman, Arthur Kleinman, John Lantos), but only Helman is in the practice of general medicine; Kleinman is a psychiatrist, Lantos a pediatrician. Helman writes for his fellow clinicians, but especially for medical students. Because his book contains a wealth of case studies and clinical data, particularly about the common, everyday problems patients bring to their doctors, his book is useful for anyone who wants to understand the rich culture that is seen in the daily practice of medicine.

Besides relating the theoretical to the practical, Helman also has the knack for concise definition and clear prose. In a useful introduction about the scope of medical anthropology, he discusses culture as the way we view the world and attempt to understand it. And he notes that culture must be seen in context ? one that is historical, economic, political, and social. Anthropologists, Helman points out, have developed two main approaches to their work. One is ethnographic, the small-scale study of how groups of people react to their world. The other is comparative, contrasting societies or different cultures. Obviously, medical historians should be on familiar ground here. And the practicing physician should also be both historian and ethnographer.

In *Culture, Health and Illness,*[68] Helman follows the division of health into the three overlapping sectors suggested by Arthur Kleinman: the popular sector, the domain of nonprofessional healers where much family care of illness takes place; a folk sector, large in non-Western societies, where health is usually viewed as a balance (both natural and supernatural) between people and their environment; and, finally, the professional sector, the site of legally sanctioned healing practices.

Helman's book describes the languages used by patients and healers. He explains a variety of illnesses and discusses the large topic of gender relationships, especially as they occur between doctors and patients in the area of reproduction. In other chapters Helman describes the many ways of responding to pain, the cultural influences on the use of drugs for treating the sick, and the various causes of and responses to the stresses of life.

He shows that cultural factors play a far more important role in all medical encounters, as well as in the epidemiology of health and disease, than a close adherence to the highly touted biomedical model. His unusual book is full of good examples, along with a clinical and social wisdom derived from a wide outlook and years of experience. These qualities make it a candidate for required reading by all of our medical students. For medical historians, as I have already indicated, Helman's book provides a rich series of examples and plentiful analytic and descriptive material about medical tasks.

Evolutionary Theory

One of the anthropological books for our review is *Evolution of Sickness and Healing* by Horacio Fabrega, a psychiatrist and anthropologist who has written about ethnomedicine since the 1970s.[86,87] Fabrega's most recent book is difficult reading, but it makes a good case for using evolutionary theory to synthesize the social, cultural, and biological aspects of health and healing. His book brings us to the last general theme that we may see in some of the more recent books about the history of medicine writ large—the new emphasis on what has been called Darwinian medicine.

Evolutionary biology, known even before Darwin's book on natural selection in 1859,[88] has not played much of a role in medical thought in the twentieth century. It was a long article by an evolutionary biologist, George C. Williams, and a psychiatrist, Randolph M. Nesse, published in the *Quarterly Review of Biology* in 1991, that once again called attention to what they called "The Dawn of Darwinian Medicine."[89]

Evolutionary biology, these authors noted in their landmark article, played virtually no role in the medical curriculum—nor, we might add, does it in the biology courses now taught in most colleges and universities. Williams and Nesse called attention to the mechanism of adaptation in understanding and treating diseases resulting from injury, infection, toxic agents, and genetic factors. Such commonly encountered medical problems as fever, pain, and swelling, and the nausea associated with early pregnancy, may all be important adaptive mechanisms to protect the body. These adaptations, the authors point out, were probably designed for stone-age life, not the environment of our time. Physicians need to view reactions to injury and disease in Darwinian terms, Williams and Nesse stress, lest their treatments harm rather than help. It has been shown, for instance, that a decrease in circulating iron is helpful in overcoming some infections. And the routine prescription of antidiarrheal medicines in cases of shigella infection actually increases the rate of complications and slows recovery.

Williams and Nesse claim that we are only at the dawn of a Darwinian medicine, even though the Darwinian theory of evolution has been a foundation of biology for nearly a century and a half. Why, then, are medicine and biology once again paying more attention to evolution? One intriguing hypothesis they offer is that, "the delay resulted mainly because scientific medicine arose during the heyday of logical positivism and its condemnation of all implications of purpose."[90] Whether a more extensive historical study will substantiate this claim remains to be seen. What is clear, however, is that here again we see the history of medicine writ large.

In their 1994 book *Why We Get Sick: The New Science of Darwinian Medicine,*[91] Nesse and Williams greatly expand the argument and the data, and spell out the implications of Darwinian medicine for medical education, public policy, and clinical practice. On the back cover of the paperback edition Richard Dawkins urges us to "buy two copies and give one to your doctor."

Another leading voice in this new Darwinian approach to medicine is Paul Ewald, professor of biology at Amherst College. His work has received wide coverage in the press, and his 1994 book, *Evolution of Infectious Disease,*[92] has become a standard reference. An evolutionary biologist, Christopher Wills, has written *Yellow Fever, Black Goddess: The Coevolution of People and Plagues,* in which he describes the history of yellow fever, cholera, syphilis, and AIDS in evolutionary terms.[93] More recently three professors of anthropology have edited *Evolutionary Medicine,*[94] and Edward J. Larson's *Summer for the Gods: The Scopes Trial and America's Continuing Debate Over Science and Religion* won the Pulitzer Prize for history.[95] (Even so, the State of Kansas wants to continue to teach creationism, with the blessings of major political candidates who wish to offend no one.)

Whether Darwinian medicine will be a continuing intellectual force remains to be seen. Good preventive advice based upon Darwinian principles should be far more widely dispensed by doctors, according to Nesse and Williams. "What a terrible irony and frightening harbinger it is," they conclude, "that such a noble and practical proposal to improve human health has to be couched in a way to save money," as it is in managed care.[96] As Ewald, and Williams and Nesse, have pointed out, Darwinian medicine views health and disease from a population perspective. In contrast, much of our medical teaching is still tied to a case-by-case method. Schools of public health have for years urged a population-based medicine upon us, but the fruits of biomedicine have made us victims of our own success.

Conclusion

What, finally, we may ask, can one learn from these thirty or so books, only a few of the many in medical anthropology and literary theory that have appeared in the last decade? First, they have helped the field of medical history to greatly broaden its appeal, and expand its style and its imaginative use of sources. We do indeed tell many stories and use many narrative strategies to tell them. To overlook books such as these from our sister fields would be to miss much of what has given our own field a wider perspective and greater sophistication. What it means, then, is that the paths to knowledge and understanding are varied.

The history of medicine has always been, by its very combination of history and medicine, an interdisciplinary endeavor. Thus, we should welcome those colleagues from anthropology and literary studies. This does not mean we should not uphold our own standards of scholarship as defined by our own needs and backgrounds. If we fail to take note of the fact that an increasing number of scholars in neighboring fields are incorporating the history of medicine into their own work, we may wake up one day to find that "we" have been taken over by "them," not so farfetched an idea when we stop to realize that there are far more of "them" than there are of "us."

In his recent book, *Guns, Germs, and Steel,* the physiologist Jared Diamond asks, "How can students of human history profit from the experience of scientist in other historical sciences?"[97] His answer is that historians have much to learn from the use of comparative methods and from the results of natural experiments. From the examples of the two groups of books I have discussed, I hope it has become clear that we do have available to us a very wide set of resources from which we can collect our data. In other words, we are all multidisciplinarians, now. Since it is particularly the younger historians who are working across boundaries, it seems safe to predict that the trend will continue.

There remains one last concern, having to do with our natural constituency, namely, medical students and doctors. Are we losing them? Does our historical work continue to speak to their needs and interests? Our work is not at all about telling these groups what they want to hear. It is about speaking to the problems they face and appealing to their natural intellectual curiosity. Common sense tells us that when we call all male physicians "phallocentric, patriarchal oppressors," they will go elsewhere to learn about their historical roots—or worse, will ignore them altogether. Since the art and science of medicine are eminently historical endeavors, there is history in medicine as well as history of medicine. But, I believe it will take a wider, more interdisciplinary perspective to tell that history of medicine in a way that will have meaning for medical students and doctors.

More than seventy years ago, at the dedication of the Welch Medical Library and my department at Johns Hopkins, Harvey Cushing spoke about the binding influence of a medical library on a subdividing profession. More and more, he lamented, the professor in the preclinical departments had less and less to do with medicine and medical practitioners. With a wary eye he surveyed the new chair in the history of medicine to be occupied by his venerable friend William Henry Welch. Cushing asked, on that dedicatory occasion, whether this new chair and department would "merely mean still another group of specialists having their own societies, organs of publication, separate places of meeting, separate congresses, national and international, and who will also incline to hold aloof from the army of doctors made and in the making."[98]

This was a prescient warning, one I believe we should again heed in the years ahead. There is a real place for teaching the humanities in the medical setting. Those who will be responsible for doing so will need not only to read widely in the literature of history, anthropology, and literary studies, but will also need to understand how medicine is learned, taught, and practiced if they are going to meet the needs of the army of doctors, made and in the making.

References

1. Bliss, M. *William Osler, A Life in Medicine.* Toronto, Toronto University Press, 1999.
2. Osler, W. *The Evolution of Modern Medicine.* New Haven, CT, Yale University Press, 1922, p. 218.
3. King, L. *Why Not Say It Clearly. A Guide to Scientific Writing.* Boston, Little, Brown, 1978.

4. MacDonald, M. "Anthropological Perspectives on the History of Science and Medicine." In *Information Sources in the History of Science and Medicine*, Pietro Corsi and Paul Weindling, (Eds.) London, Butterworths, 1983, pp. 61-80.
5. Ibid., p. 61.
6. Ibid., p. 62.
7. Good, B. *Medicine, Rationality, and Experience, An Anthropological Perspective.* New York, Cambridge University Press, 1994, p. 4.
8. Foster, G. and Anderson, B. *Medical Anthropology.* New York, John Wiley & Sons, 1978. See also the extensive collection of papers in David Landy, (Ed.), *Culture, Disease, and Healing: Studies in Medical Anthropology.* New York, Macmillan, 1977.
9. Comaroff, J. & J. Comaroff. *Ethnography and the Historical Imagination.* Boulder, CO, Westview Press, 1992.
10. Brieger, G.H. "Arrowsmith and the History of Medicine," *Mobius*, 2: 32-38, 1982.
11. Nussbaum, M. *Love's Knowledge: Essays on Philosophy and Literature.* New York, Oxford University Press, 1990, p 47.
12. Op. cit. #10, Brieger, p. 38.
13. Atwood, M. "In Search of *Alias Grace:* On Writing Canadian Historical Fiction," *American Historical Review,* 103: 1503, 1998.
14. Morantz-Sanchez, R. *Conduct Unbecoming to a Woman: Medicine on Trial in Turn-of-the-Century Brooklyn.* New York, Oxford University Press, 1999.
15. Geertz, C. "Blurred Genres: The Reconfiguration of Social Thought," *American Scholar,* Spring, 1980, reprinted in Geertz, *Local Knowledge: Further Essays in Interpretive Anthropology.* New York, Basic Books, 1983.
16. Brandt, Allan M. and Rozin, Paul, (Eds.). *Morality and Health.* New York, Routledge, 1997.
17. Gieryn, T.E. "Boundary-Work and the Demarcation of Science from Non-Science," *American Sociological Review,* 48: 781-95, 1983.
18. Hunter, K.M. "Narrative." In *Encyclopedia of Bioethics.* Warren Reich, (Ed.), 5 vols. New York, Macmillan, vol. 4, 1995, p. 1789
19. Epstein, J. *Altered Conditions: Disease, Medicine, and Storytelling.* New York, Routledge, 1995.
20. Bailin, M. *The Sickroom in Victorian Fiction: The Art of Being Ill.* Cambridge Studies in Nineteenth-Century Literature, No. 1. Cambridge, U.K., Cambridge University Press, 1994.
21. Vrettos, A. *Somatic Fictions: Imagining Illness in Victorian Culture.* Stanford, CA, Stanford University Press, 1995.
22. Op. cit. #19, Epstein, J., p. 17.
23. Ibid., p. 19.
24. Fissell, M. "The Disappearance of the Patient's Narrative and the Interven-

tion of Hospital Medicine." In *British Medicine in an Age of Reform,* Roger French and Andrew Wear (Eds.). London, Routledge, 1991, pp. 92-109.
25. Frank, A.W. *The Wounded Storyteller: Body, Illness and Ethics.* Chicago, University of Chicago Press, 1995.
26. Hawkins, A.H. *Reconstructing Illness: Studies in Pathography*. 2nd ed. West Lafayette, IN., Purdue University Press, 1999
27. Herndl, D.P. *Invalid Women: Figuring Feminine Illness in American Fiction and Culture.* Chapel Hill, University of North Carolina Press, 1993.
28. Showalter, Elaine. *Hystories: Hysterical Epidemics and Modern Media.* New York, Columbia University Press, 1997.
29. Furst, L.R. *Between Doctors and Patients: The Changing Balance of Power.* Charlottesville, University Press of Virginia, 1998.
30. Dixon, E.H. *Woman and Her Diseases, from the Cradle to the Grave; Adapted Exclusively to Her Construction in the Physiology of Her Systems and All the Diseases of Her Critical Period.* New York, Ring, 1847.
31 Clarke, E.H. *Sex in Education*. Boston, J.R. Osgood, 1873.
32. Jacobi, M. P. *The Question of Rest for Women During Menstruation.* 1876.
33. Wood, M.E. *The Writing on the Wall: Women's Autobiography and the Asylum.* Urbana, University of Illinois Press, 1994.
34. Howells, W.D. *Dr. Breen's Practice; a novel.* Boston, Houghton Mifflin, 1881, (reprinted Westport, CT, Greenwood Press, 1969.)
35. Phelps, E.S. *Dr. Zay,* New York, Feminist Press at the City University of New York, 1987.
36. Jewett, S.O. *A Country Doctor,* New York, New American Library, 1986.
37. James, H. *The Bostonians,* New York, Modern Library, 1956.
38. Nathan-Meyer, A. *Helen Brent, M.D.,* New York, Cassell, 1892. Reproduction: Woodbridge, CT, Reseaarch Publications, 1970-1978.
39. Burns, C.R. "Fictional Doctors and the Evolution of Medical Ethics in the United States, 1875 – 1900," *Literature and Medicine*, 7: 39-55, 1998.
40. Porter, R. "Introduction," in Peter Logan, *Nerves and Narratives: A Cultural History of Hysteria in Nineteenth-Century British Prose.* Berkeley and Los Angeles, University of California Press, 1997.
41. Arnold, D. *Colonizing the Body, State Medicine and Epidemic Disease in Nineteenth-Century India.* Berkeley and Los Angeles, University of California Press, 1993, p. 9.
42. Wolf, N. *The Beauty Myth: How Images of Beauty Are Used Against Women.* New York, Anchor Books, 1991.
43. Brumberg, J. *The Body Project: An Intimate History of American Girls.* New York, Random House, 1997.
44. Haiken, E. *Venus Envy: A History of Cosmetic Surgery*. Baltimore, Johns Hopkins University Press, 1997.
45. Gilman, S. *Making The Body Beautiful: A Cultural History of Aesthetic*

Surgery. Princeton, NJ, Princeton University Press, 1999.
46. Gilman, S. *The Jew's Body.* New York, Routledge, 1991.
47. Lay, M.M., Gurak, L.J., Gravon, C., & Myntia, C. (Eds.). *Body Talk: Rhetoric, Technology, Reproduction.* Madison, University of Wisconsin Press, 2000.
48. Scheper-Hughes, N. and Lock, M.M. "The Mindful Body: A Prolegomenon to Future Work in Medical Anthropology," *Medical Anthropology Quarterly*, 1: 6-41, 1987.
49. Porter, R. "History of the Body," in *New Perspectives on Historical Writing.* Peter Burke (Ed.). University Park, Pennsylvania State University Press, 1992, pp. 206-32.
50. Logan, P.M. *Nerves and Narratives: A Cultural History of Hysteria in Nineteenth-Century British Prose.* Berkeley and Los Angeles, University of California Press, 1997. p. 11.
51. Poovey, M. *Making A Social Body: British Cultural Formation,* 1830-1864. Chicago, University of Chicago Press, 1995.
52. Chadwick, E. Sanitary Condition of the Labouring Population of Great Britain, 1842. National Library of Medicine, HMD Collection, Call number WAAG 786r 1842.
53. Otis, L. *Membranes: Metaphors of Invasion in Nineteenth-Century Literature, Science, and Politics.* Baltimore, Johns Hopkins University Press, 1999.
54. Murphy, R. in *Disability and Culture,* Benedicte Ingstad and Susan Reynolds Whyte (Eds.). Berkeley and Los Angeles: University of California Press, 1995, p. 140.
55. Goffman, E. *Stigma: Notes on the Management of Spoiled Identity.* Englewood Cliffs, NJ, Prentice Hall [1963].
56. Thomson, R.G. *Extraordinary Bodies: Figuring Physical Disability in American Culture and Literature.* New York, Columbia University Press, 1997.
57. Stowe, H.B. *Uncle Tom's Cabin.* New York: Literary Classics of the U.S.: Distributed by the Viking Press, 1982.
58. Davis, R.H. *Life in the Iron Mills and Other Stories,* edited with a biographical interpretation by T. Olsen, Old Westbury, New York, Feminist Press, 1985.
59. Phelps, E.S. *The Silent Partner,* Ridgewood, NJ, Gregg Press, 1967.
60. Mitchell, D.T. and S.L. Snyder (Eds.). *The Body and Physical Difference: Discourses of Disability. The Body in Theory: Histories of Cultural Materialism*. Ann Arbor, University of Michigan Press, 1997.
61. Yuan, D.D. Disfigurement and reconstruction in Oliver Wendell Holmes' 'The Human Wheel, the Spokes and Felloes.' Op. cit. #60, pp. 71-88.
62. Molina, C. Muteness and Mutilation: The Aesthetics of Disability in Jane

Campion's *The Piano*. Op. cit. #60, pp. 267-282.

63. Ingstad, B. and S.R. Whyte (Eds.). *Disability and Culture.* Berkeley and Los Angeles, University of California Press, 1995.
64. Morris, D. *The Culture of Pain.* Berkeley and Los Angeles: University of California Press, 1991.
65. Kleinman, A., Das, V., and Lock, M. (Eds.). *Social Suffering.* Berkeley and Los Angeles, University of California Press, 1997.
66. Ibid. p. ix.
67. Ibid. p. 9.
68. Helman, C.G. (Ed.). *Culture, Health, and Illness: An Introduction for Health Professionals.* 3rd ed. Oxford, Butterworth-Heinemann, 1997.
69. Kleinman, A. *Writing at the Margin: Discourse between Anthropology and Medicine.* Berkeley and Los Angeles, University of California Press, 1995.
70. Hahn, R. *Sickness and Healing, An Anthropological Perspective.* New Haven, CT, Yale University Press, 1995.
71. Stein, H.F. *American Medicine as Culture.* Boulder, CO, Westview Press, 1990.
72. Good, B.J. *Medicine, Rationality, and Experience: An Anthropological Perspective.* New York, Cambridge University Press, 1994.
73. Good, M.D. *American Medicine: The Quest for Competence.* Berkeley and Los Angeles, University of California Press, 1995.
74. Good, B.J. and M.J.D. Good. Learning Medicine, The Construction of Medical Knowledge at Harvard Medical School. In: *Knowledge, Power and Practice: The Anthropology of Medicine and Everyday Life,* S. Lindenbaurn and M. Lock (Eds.). Berkeley and Los Angeles, University of California Press, 1993.
75. Tosteson, D.C., S.J. Adelstein, and S.I Carver (Eds.). *New Pathways to Medical Education: Learning to Learn at Harvard Medical School.* Cambridge, MA, Harvard University Press, 1994.
76. Merton, R.K., G. Reader, and P.L. Kendall (Eds.). *The Student Physician, Introductory Studies in the Sociology of Medical Education.* Cambridge, MA, Harvard University Press, 1957.
77. Becker, H.S., B. Geer, E.C. Hughes, and A.L. Strauss. *Boys in White, Student Culture in Medical School.* Chicago, University of Chicago Press, 1961.
78. Op. cit. #73, Good and Good, p. 98.
79. Ibid., p. 103.
80. Hawkins, A.H. and M.C. McEntyre (Eds.). *Teaching Literature and Medicine.* Modern Language Association of America Options for Teaching. New York, Modern Language Association, 2000.
81. Coles, R. *The Call of Stories: Teaching and the Moral Imagination.* Boston, Houghton Mifflin, 1989.

82. Brody, H. *Stories of Sickness.* New Haven, CT, Yale University Press, 1988.
83. Hunter, K.M. *Doctor's Stories: The Narrative Structure of Medical Knowledge.* Princeton, NJ, Princeton University Press, 1991.
84. See also G.S. Rousseau, "Literature and Medicine: The State of the Field," *Isis*, 72: 406-24, 1981; Rita Charon, "Doctor-Patient, Reader-Writer: Learning to Find the Text," *Soundings,* 72: 137-52, 1989; and Rita Charon et al., "Literature and Medicine: Contributions to Clinical Practice," *Annals of Internal Medicine,* 122: 599-606, 1995.
85. Osler, W. *The Evolution of Modern Medicine.* New Haven, CT, Yale University Press, 1922, p. 218.
86. See especially Fabrega's widely cited "The Need for an Ethno-Medical Science," *Science,* 189: 969-75, 1975.
87. Fabrega, H. Jr. *Evolution of Sickness and Healing.* Berkeley and Los Angeles, University of California Press, 1997.
88. Darwin, C. *On the Origins of Species by Means of Natural Selection or the Preservation of Favored Races in the Struggle for Life.* London, Murray, 1859.
89. Williams, G.C. and R.M. Nesse. "The Dawn of Darwinian Medicine." *Quarterly Review of Biology,* 66: 1-22, 1991.
90. Ibid., p. 17.
91. Nesse, R. M. and G.C. Williams. *Why We Get Sick: The New Science of Darwinian Medicine.* New York, Random House, 1995. p. 248.
92. Ewald, P.W. *Evolution of Infectious Disease.* New York, Oxford University Press, 1994.
93. Wills, C. *Yellow Fever, Black Goddess: The Coevolution of People and Plagues.* Reading, MA, Addison-Wesley, 1996.
94. Trevathan, W.R., E.D. Smith, and J.J. McKenna (Eds.). *Evolutionary Medicine.* New York, Oxford University Press, 1999.
95. Larson, E.S. *Summer for the Gods: The Scopes Trial and America's Continuing Debate Over Science and Religion.* Cambridge, MA, Harvard University Press, 1997.
96. Ibid., p. 248.
97. Diamond, J. *Guns, Germs and Steel: The Fates of Human Societies.* New York, Norton, 1997, p. 424.
98. Cushing, H. "The Binding Influence On a Subdividing Profession." *Bulletin of The Johns Hopkins Hospital,* 46: 38, 1930.

Selected Readings

The following list of books are those included in two essay reviews for the *Bulletin of the History of Medicine.* Not all of these books are discussed in the McGovern Lecture.

Vincanne Adams. *Doctors for Democracy: Health Professionals in the Nepal Revolution.* Cambridge, U.K., Cambridge University Press, 1998.

H. E Augstein. James Cowles Prichard's Anthropology: Remaking the Science of Man in Early Nineteenth Century Britain. Clio Medica, Vol. 52. Wellcome Institute Series in the History of Medicine. Amsterdam: Editions Rodopi, 1999.

David Bevan (Ed.). *Literature and Sickness.* Rodopi Perspectives on Modern Literature, no. 8. Amsterdam: Rodopi, 1993.

Ellen Messer-Davidow, David R. Shurnway, and David J. Sylvain (Eds.). *Knowledges: Historical and Critical Studies in Disciplinarity.* Charlottesville: University of Virginia Press, 1993.

Carl Elliott and John Lantos (Eds.). *The Last Physician: Walker Percy and the Moral Life of Medicine.* Durham, NC: Duke University Press, 1999.

Lilian R. Furst. *Just Talk: Narratives of Psychotherapy.* Lexington: University Press of Kentucky, 1999.

Susan C. Greenfield and Carol Barash (Eds.). *Inventing Maternity: Politics, Science and Literature, 1650 - 1865.* Lexington: University of Kentucky Press, 1999.

Roslynn D. Hayes. *From Faust to Strangelove: Representations of the Scientist in Western Literature.* Baltimore: Johns Hopkins University Press, 1994.

Cecil G. Helman, Thomas M. Johnson and Carolyn E Sargeant (Eds.). *Medical Anthropology: Contemporary Theory and Method.* New York: Praeger, 1990.

Jens Lachmund and Gunnar Stollberg (Eds.). *The Social Construction of Illness. Medizin, Gesellschaft, und Geschichte,* Suppl 1 . Stuttgart: Franz Steiner Verlag, *1992.*

John D. Lantos. *Do We Still Need Doctors?* Reflective Bioethics series. New York: Routledge, 1997.

Margaret Lock and Deborah Gordon (Eds.). *Biomedicine Examined.* Dordrecht: Kluwer Academic Publishers, 1988.

David B. Morris. *Illness and Culture in the Postmodern Age.* Berkeley and Los Angeles: University of California Press, 1998.

Phillip A. Scott. *The Medical Research Novel in English and German, 1900-1950.* Bowling Green, Ohio: Bowling Green State University Popular Press, 1992.

Simon Sinclair. *Making Doctors: An Institutional Apprenticeship.* Explorations in Anthropology. New York: New York University Press, 1997.

Helen Small. *Love's Madness: Medicine, the Novel, and Female Insanity, 1800-1865.* Oxford: Clarendon Press, 1996.

Delese Wear and Lois LaCivita Nixon. *Literary Anatomies: Women's Bodies and Health in Literature.* Albany: State University of New York Press, 1994.

Allan Young. The Harmony of Illusions: Inventing Post-Traumatic Stress Disorder. Princeton, NJ: Princeton University Press, 1995.

Reflections on American Medical Education*

Kenneth M. Ludmerer

Kenneth M. Ludmerer is Professor of Medicine in the School of Medicine and Professor of History in the Faculty of Arts and Sciences at Washington University, St. Louis. A native of Long Beach, California, he received an A.B. from Harvard College and an M.A. and M.D. from The Johns Hopkins University School of Medicine. Following medical school, he did graduate work in history at Harvard and a residency in internal medicine at Barnes Hospital in St. Louis, after which he joined the faculty of Washington University.

Dr. Ludmerer is best known for his work in medical education and the history of medicine. He has written three books: *Genetics and American Society* (1972), a study of the American eugenics movement; *Learning to Heal* (1985), which details the creation of America's system of medical education, and *Time to Heal* (1999), an examination of the evolution of American medical education from the turn of the Twentieth Century to the present age of managed care. Reviewers have called the latter book "a masterpiece of great national importance" and "the most important work in medical education since the Flexner report."

Dr. Ludmerer is a member of numerous professional organizations including Phi Beta Kappa, Alpha Omega Alpha, the Association of American Physicians, and the American Clinical and Climatological Association, and the American Academy of Arts and Sciences. He is President of the American Association for the History of Medicine (2002-2004), past-president of the American Osler Society (1994-1995), and a member of the National Council of Harvard Medical School. His awards include the Nicholas E. Davies Award of

*Delivered 18 April 2001 at the Thirty-first Annual Meeting of the American Osler Society, Charleston, South Carolina.

the American College of Physicians for Outstanding Contributions to the Medical Humanities (1997); the Distinguished Alumnus Award of the Johns Hopkins University (2000); the inaugural Daniel C. Tosteson Award for Leadership in Medical Education from Harvard Medical School's Carl J. Shapiro Institute (2001).

It is a great privilege to have the opportunity to deliver the sixteenth John P. McGovern Award Lectureship to the American Osler Society. Dr. McGovern is not only an important member and great friend of this organization, but a leader of American medicine and an exemplary medical humanist as well. The American Osler Society is a very special organization—for the values it exemplifies, the quality of its papers and discussions, and the camaraderie of its membership. I was totally surprised to be asked to deliver this lecture, given that McGovern Lecturers typically come from outside the society, but that makes this honor even more meaningful to me.

For all William Osler's accomplishments and attributes, above all he was a teacher and educator. Among his contributions, he championed the importance of the inductive method of medical education ("learning by doing"), and introduced the clinical clerkship to American medical schools. Now that we are at the beginning of a new century, we have a suitable opportunity to review the major challenges and obstacles that medical education presently faces.

In this lecture I wish to focus on two types of challenges to medical education. First, I shall review the major "internal" challenges to medical education. By this I mean the obstacles to medical teaching that have arisen from the internal intellectual development of medical knowledge and practice. Then, I shall discuss the critical "external" challenges that medical education faces at the present moment. By "external," I mean threats to medical education that have arisen from changes in American society and the health care delivery system. My observations are drawn from the two books on medical education I have written, *Learning to Heal* [1] and *Time to Heal,* [2] as well as from reflections on the response to *Time to Heal* during the past year.

Internal Challenges

The first internal issue pertains to the challenges to medical teaching posed by the molecular revolution in biomedical science. For most of the twentieth century, a distinctive feature of medical education in the United States was the integration of research with teaching and patient care. The cohesiveness between teaching and research was made possible because instructors taught students what they themselves were investigating. However, as biomedical research after 1970 became increasingly molecular in its intellectual orientation, teachers found it increasingly difficult to be cutting-edge researchers, and vice versa. Accordingly, the identification of teachers, both in the scientific and clinical disciplines, became a difficult task.

Today, this difficulty is especially clear in the basic science fields, where the research interests of most faculty no longer directly relate to much of the subject matter still taught to medical students. Professors in these fields are in the awkward position of studying fundamental molecular and cellular biology, for which they are rewarded, while teaching clinically necessary subjects they do not particularly value, such as gross and microscopic anatomy, fluid and electrolyte metabolism, and classic organ physiology. In some fields, it has become difficult to find faculty who can still teach the classical subject matter. Gross anatomy is the prime example. Anatomy departments now depend heavily on surgeons, radiologists, anthropologists, and dentists for help in teaching, since the field is virtually dead as an area of active investigation among anatomy faculty (most of whom now work in cell biology). To a lesser extent, this problem affects instruction in the other basic science departments as well. At the dawn of the twenty-first century, officials at some schools are acknowledging the possibility that the basic science departments might be forced to split into separate research and teaching faculties.

Similar developments have occurred in the clinical departments, where the traditional cohesiveness among research, patient care, and education has substantially eroded. Until around 1970, the defining characteristic of clinical research was its focus upon patients. This meant that clinical research went hand-in-hand with patient care and clinical instruction. In the molecular era, patients have been bypassed in clinical research. The results of this approach have been gratifying in terms of medical discovery. However, for the first time, a conspicuous separation of functions has occurred between clinical research and clinical teaching.

Clinical departments at many schools have responded by establishing two faculty tracks: a "clinician-teacher" track for faculty concentrating on education and patient care, and an "academic track" for laboratory investigators. Most faculty members specializing in "evidence-based medicine" have joined the clinical track because of their familiarity with the clinical literature and their expertise in delivering medical care. However, such an approach merely highlights the fundamental problem it was meant to solve: the growing estrangement between teaching and research. Experts in evidence-based medicine seldom possess the clinical investigator's knowledge of the molecular mechanisms of disease and therapeutics, while today's clinical investigators are much more removed from day-to-day patient care and clinical teaching than clinical professors in the past. In the clinical departments, as in the basic science departments, no one has a good answer to the vexing question, "Who are the teachers?"

A second internal obstacle to creating a rich educational environment is the traditional tension at U.S. medical schools between teaching and research. The

American medical school, like the American research university, was created by scholars for scholars. This has resulted in an institutional culture that rewards research accomplishments far more than educational effectiveness. Medical schools have long uttered much lip service about the importance of the educational mission. However, their actions have not confirmed their words, as all century long they have granted promotions and other institutional rewards mainly for research, not teaching. Indeed, the folklore of academic medicine has long held that the sure way for an instructor not to be promoted is to win an award for good teaching.

The emphasis on research was not intrinsically harmful to medical education. Indeed, throughout the twentieth century educators have commonly maintained that research invigorated teaching, by enabling a scholarly atmosphere for the study of medicine. Students were exposed to the reasoning skills of the finest medical minds, and they became aware of the tentative nature of even the seemingly most secure pieces of medical knowledge. The presence of research kept medical education from going overboard teaching practical details instead of fundamental principles, and reminded educators that students needed time to think, digest, and wonder.

Nevertheless, there was also an intrinsic conflict between teaching and research: they competed for a faculty member's time. Teaching, when done well, was time-consuming and labor-intensive, requiring close personal contact with students. Good teaching required a generalist and synthetic orientation that in an era of increasing specialization took greater and greater effort to provide. Herein lay the primary obstacle medical schools encountered in trying to improve their educational programs: time spent teaching meant less time for research. It was difficult to entice faculty members to give much attention to students when they were seldom rewarded by the institution for doing so. Hence the frequent neglect of teaching, whether at the medical school or the research university.

As a result, for the past century medical schools have evolved in a faculty-centered, not a student-centered, manner. In the basic science subjects, the domination of the curriculum by lectures and the de-emphasis of laboratories and individualized instruction represented a much more efficient use of faculty time. In the clinical subjects, the use of house officers as teaching assistants served a similar purpose; freeing the faculty to pursue their other interests, particularly research. By their actions, medical schools everywhere demonstrated a widespread lack of concern for student matters: the difficulty in recruiting faculty to serve on admissions committees or to help with interviews, repeated complaints from students that they were neglected, reports of the unavailability of faculty advisers, the behavior of faculty who resented their lecture duties (for instance, delivering their lectures without introducing themselves to the class), the refusal of departmental chairpersons to sit on curriculum committees, the conversion of student teaching laboratories into faculty research laboratories, the unwillingness of some faculty to write letters of recommendations for students, and poor faculty turnouts at commencement exercises. This deeply ingrained subordination of teaching to research in the value system of U.S. medical schools has presented a formidable obstacle to medical education all century long.

A third internal issue is the relative lack of preparation of today's students for the management of patients with chronic diseases. Medical educators created the hospital clerkship, the mainstay of clinical education, in the late nineteenth century, when life expectancy in the U.S. was barely forty years and when acute illnesses (infections, injuries, and acute manifestations of chronic diseases) dominated medical practice. Today, as a result of the success of public health and modern medicine, life expectancy in the U.S. is approaching eighty years, and chronic and degenerative diseases dominate the practices of most physicians.

The diagnosis and management of chronic diseases, unlike that of many acute illnesses, is largely an outpatient activity. During the past two decades, there have been many calls for medical schools to provide more and better ambulatory experiences, so that students might obtain greater exposure to patients with chronic illnesses. The Association of American Medical College's "GPEP" Report in 1984[3] was the most prominent of these calls. Nevertheless, on balance, medical schools continue to rely on inpatient hospital clerkships for the great majority of clinical instruction. How students are to acquire the knowledge, skills, and attitudes required for the care of patients with chronic diseases is a conspicuous deficiency in medical education today. It remains uncertain whether current students will be fully prepared for many of the most important challenges they are likely to face when they begin the practice of medicine.

External Challenges

Throughout the twentieth century, American medical schools have found themselves with two homes: one in the university, the other in the health care delivery system. Of the two, the ties to the university have traditionally been far stronger. Since the passage of the Medicare and Medicaid legislation in 1965, the patient care activities of medical faculties have grown enormously, and the ties of the medical schools to the health care delivery system have correspondingly increased. Accordingly, academic medical centers are now firmly enmeshed in the health care delivery system—and hence subject to all the forces and cross currents of this system. In the current environment, this has led to a series of unprecedented "external" threats, both to academic medical centers as institutions and to the quality of medical education they are able to provide.

The most obvious consequence of today's market-driven health care environment for academic medical centers is financial. Because of education, research, charity care, and a sicker case mix of patients, the costs of teaching hospitals run about 25 to 30 percent higher than those of community hospitals. Previously, third-party payers were willing to accept higher bills from teaching hospitals to cross-subsidize these socially important activities. In the 1990s, however, insurers were increasingly unwilling to do so. Instead, they insisted on paying only for the costs of hospital care actually incurred by their enrollees. Accordingly, the margins teaching institutions depended on for education and research were whittled away. In 2000, the University of Pennsylvania Health System—one of the country's strongest and best medical centers—suffered a $200,000,000 operating loss. It has been estimated that if current trends go unchecked, as many as two-thirds of teaching centers will be operating in the red within five years. Academic medical centers now find themselves in a buyers' market indifferent to their needs—a market where insurers are rapidly withdrawing from the support of socially valuable functions they had nurtured for over half a century.

From the educational perspective, many of the current difficulties of medical education have arisen from the responses of teaching institutions to these financial pressures. In general, academic medical centers have responded to the lower payments they are receiving by increasing the volume of patients they see. By caring for enough patients fast enough, they hope to remain solvent, at least for the moment. Such behavior, though understandable from a purely business perspective, has come at a great price: academic medical centers have begun to lose sight of their mission and *raison d'être*. Institutional survival is being accomplished, but in the process the core principles those institutions have been entrusted to preserve are being sacrificed. Today, academic medical centers are rapidly losing their academic qualities, and the opportunities for students and house officers to acquire fundamental clinical skills and caring attitudes have been seriously undermined.

The market's erosive effects on medical education are exerted in many ways. For instance, fewer and fewer clinical faculty are available to serve as teachers and mentors. Instead, today's faculty are under intense pressure to be "clinically productive"—that is, to see as many paying patients as possible so that they can help keep the medical center financially afloat. (The common definition of "clinical productivity" at medical schools refers to the amount of professional fees generated, not to the quantity or quality of care. Delivering ordinary care to paying patients is considered clinically productive; delivering outstanding care to charity patients is not.) This writer knows of a chairman of internal medicine at a prestigious medical school who has told his faculty, "If you want to teach, do so at lunch—and keep your lunches short." Because of such pressures, many clinical faculty presently have little time to teach, advise, serve as mentors, or conduct research. In addition, medical students' opportunities to observe faculty doctoring in a teacherly, caring way are dwindling. If there was one tenet of medical education that helped to ensure medicine's place as a university discipline in the twentieth century, it was the importance of conducting medical education in a scholarly environment. This principle is being violated by the shift in emphasis from teaching and research to patient care, and by the conversion of a scholarly faculty into an exclusively clinical faculty.

Though teachers are important to the learning environment, the opportunity for students to spend ample time with patients is even more critical. In this respect, the marketplace has again been extremely injurious to clinical learning. Through the mid-1980s, the average length of stay at teaching hospitals was ten to twelve days. Now, it is three to four days. In part this change reflects technological advances in medical care, such as the growing use of minimally invasive surgery. However, it largely represents the attempt by third-party payers to reduce hospital costs. Short hospital stays have forced medical schools to conduct clinical education in an atmosphere in which speed is the principal mandate for patient care. As a result, students are being converted from active learners to passive observers, with deleterious consequences for their ability to acquire fundamental knowledge and skills.

Among the negative effects of today's clinical environment on the education of students is its impact on the acquisition of cognitive skills. It is much harder for learners to develop problem-solving abilities when patients are admitted with their diagnoses known and treatment plans already determined. Clinical clerks in surgery, meeting patients under the drapes of the operating table, can still learn about removing a gall bladder, but such encounters do not teach students to recognize the patients who might actually need the procedure from those who do not. Once admitted, patients are often discharged before a diagnosis has been made or the effects of therapy observed—even before an attending physician has had the chance to confirm a physical finding. These circumstances deprive students of the opportunity to follow the course of disease and treatment.

Of equal concern are the negative implications of this hurried environment for the all-important latent learning of the "hidden curriculum." Habits of thoroughness, attentiveness to detail, questioning, and listening are difficult to instill when learning occurs in a clinical environment more strongly committed to patient "throughput" than to patient satisfaction. In addition, it is hard to imagine how caring attitudes can easily be developed when medical education is conducted in a highly commercial atmosphere where a good visit is a short visit, patients are "consumers," and institutional officials speak more often of the financial balance sheet than of the relief of suffering.

Thus, as the twenty-first century begins, the university system that characterized American medical education during the twentieth century is being taken apart, and a second revolutionary period in American medical education is starting. The challenge of the first revolution in medical education was to pull medical education from the environment of medical practice into the university. Now, medical educators are raising the question whether medical schools should leave their universities to join integrated delivery systems. A task of the first revolution was to establish research as a major focus of the medical school. Today, medical educators often find themselves apologizing about research, and some even have asked whether the classic model of the research-intensive medical school should be allowed to persist in the future. A goal of the first revolution had been to make medical education a true university activity by freeing medical professors from having to practice medicine to make a living. Now, as at the proprietary schools a century before, clinical faculty find themselves increasingly dependent on private practice for their livelihood. A central mission of the first revolution was to create a stimulating learning environment to help assure that medical education would be graduate education rather than vocational training. At the turn of the new century, the clinical learning environment is rapidly eroding, with serious implications for the quality of medical education. During the first revolution, university presidents had taken a deep interest in medical education, and many had helped lead the movement to create a strong system of university-based medical schools. Today, few university presidents are defending medical schools' goals of education and research, and even fewer seem to be aware that medical schools are in danger of leaving the university. These comparisons could be continued, but it is clear that medical education at present is reverting toward a proprietary system that university and medical leaders had self-consciously rejected a century ago.

Solving the External Challenges

As the above discussion has shown, academic medical centers find themselves at the dawn of a new century with less self-confidence and a greater sense of loss of control than at any time in nearly a century. Yet, for advocates of quality in medical education, there is reason not to despair. The past, bearing as it always does on the present, harbors the principles by which academic medical centers and society can better serve each other so that high standards might be retained. Specific solutions will need to be crafted for the twenty-first century; tactics appropriate for one time, place, and social context typically do not serve as a template for another. However, guiding principles can be derived from an understanding of the past. The key lies in restoring the tattered social contract between society and academic medicine.

For the general public, there is one overarching message: academic medical centers are fragile institutions that need aggressive nurturing, sustained protection, and the unwavering support of those with vision, power, and means. The most important social functions of academic medical centers—the education of future generations of medical professionals, the discovery of new medical knowledge, the provision of highly specialized clinical services, and the care of poor and uninsured persons—are activities that are revenue-draining, not income-generating. Insurers and third-party payers have traditionally helped pay for these public services, but most managed care organizations are unwilling to do so. If American medicine is to retain its future-directedness and its humanity—its investment in education and research, and its capacity to serve the sickest patients and those who cannot afford to pay—specific sources of funding for the public missions of academic medical centers must be provided.

For medical educators, there is also an overarching message: external support cannot be expected without convincing demonstration that academic medical centers are serving the needs of the public. Medical schools and teaching hospitals have always existed for the community's well being, and not vice versa. Yet somehow since the 1970s, many medical faculties have forgotten this fact. If medical educators are to succeed in preserving the vitality of academic medical centers, they need to remember the admonition of Charles Eliot, a former president of Harvard University, that "the first step toward getting an endowment is to deserve one."

Medical faculties have a number of issues to address if they are to demonstrate that they are still deserving of generous public support. First, they need to adjust more fully to the new environment of resource constraints. This entails becoming leaner, more efficient, more agile, and more cost-effective in the practice of medicine. This also requires a far more effective process of long-range planning. Academic medical centers can no longer try to be all things to all people; rather, they will finally have to make tough decisions about which academic areas to pursue and which to leave to someone else. They will also have to reevaluate the optimal size of their student enrollments, graduate training programs, and faculty and support staffs. Collectively, they will even have to address the thorny question of whether the nation's medical schools and residency programs are producing too many doctors for the country's needs, and if so, how to correct the problem.

Second, medical schools needed to do a better job of producing the types of doctors that the country needs. There is a distinct need to improve instruction in such areas as cost-consciousness, preventive medicine, health promotion, ambulatory medicine, primary care, the appropriate use of diagnostic tests, and the psychological dimensions of patient care. Faculties need to accelerate the effort to introduce a population perspective into medical education—that is, to teach strategies to maximize the health of a defined population (such as that of an HMO) with the resources at hand. Faculties also need to work on those factors under their control to produce a specialty mix more closely aligned with the health care needs of the country.

Third, medical faculties can demonstrate that they are serving the public interest by regaining the critical initiative in monitoring and maintaining the quality of care, which in the view of many observers has been eroding for over a decade. The answer to preserving quality is not open-ended spending. Rather, the intellectual elite of the profession need to provide guidance regarding how to use resources wisely. If academic and professional leaders can speak in a unified voice about what is best for patients, a powerful force for the public good could be released.

Lastly, medical faculties need to make clear that their research interests are fully concordant with the health concerns of the public. In an era of chronic diseases and an aging population, this means integrating the study of the organization, financing, and delivery of health care with traditional scientific work. All the rich intellectual resources of the university could be called upon to assist in this effort. Of course, something as large and complex as the health care delivery system is not the sole responsibility of academic medicine to fix. However, the problems of promoting health and organizing health care in the United States have become so pressing that they deserve much more attention from medical schools than they have traditionally received. Certainly, rapid evolution of the country's health care system is going to continue with or without the involvement of medical educators, but without their participation, they and the public are less likely to be satisfied with the results.

Though imposing, these challenges are not as daunting as they might seem at first glance. There are many reasons to be optimistic, and the challenges of maintaining a strong system of medical education are not as great as those of creating the system a century ago. At the start of the twenty-first century the public is already accustomed to supporting medical schools generously, the capacity of medical care and potential of medical research are widely recognized, the public is expressing its belief in medicine by spending over a trillion dollars a year on health care, considerable national goodwill toward the medical profession remains, the public is realizing that managed care needs significant improvements, and the majority of physicians retain a conscience and a deep-seated sense of service. These represent major advantages not available to the pioneering medical educators and create genuine hope that the social contract might be restored. At the present moment, the time available to do so is shrinking —but there is still opportunity for visionaries to dream, for men and women of good will to stand up for principle, and for leaders to act.

References

1. Ludmerer, Kenneth M. *Learning to Heal: The Development of American Medical Education.* New York, Basic Books, 1985.
2. Ludmerer, Kenneth M. *Time to Heal: American Medical Education from the Turn of the Century to the Era of Managed Care.* New York, Oxford University Press, 1999.
3. Association of American Medical Colleges, Physicians for the twenty-first century, report of the Project Panel on the General Professional Education of the Physician and College Preparation for Medicine. *J Med Educ* 59 (11 Pt 2): i-208, 1984.

John Shaw Billings as a Historian*

James H. Cassedy

James H. Cassedy received his secondary education in Fultonville, New York, his undergraduate degree in American Literature from Middlebury College, and his doctorate in American Civilization from Brown University. After five years in the United States Army during World War II, he served in the U.S. Veterans Administration and in the U.S. Information Agency before beginning an academic career at Williams College.

In 1962, he became Executive Secretary of the History of the Life Sciences Study Section at the National Institutes of Health. He later served the National Institutes of Health as Deputy Chief of the European Office in Paris, France. Since 1968, he has been Historian at the National Library of Medicine, where he also edits the *Bibliography of the History of Medicine* and HISTLINE, and manages the History of Medicine Seminar Program. In addition to numerous articles, his books include: *Charles V. Chapin and the Public Health Movement* (1962); *Demography in Early America ...* (1969); *American Medicine and Statistical Thinking, 1800-1860* (1984); *Medicine and American Growth, 1800-1860* (1986); and *Medicine in America ...* (1991). He is currently preparing a book-length study on John Shaw Billings' influence on American medicine and public health.

Dr. Cassedy was president of the American Association for the History of Medicine 1982-1984. His avocations are reading, travel, and playing the piano.

*Delivered 24 April 2002 at the Thirty-Second Annual Meeting of the American Osler Society, Kansas City, Kansas.

Several years ago, the historian Genevieve Miller wrote a scholarly paper "in praise" of the amateur physician-historians of late nineteenth-century America. In her paper, she drew attention to a considerable number of such physicians who, working mainly in their spare time, had made significant and sometimes substantial contributions to medical history: as translators, writers, book collectors, librarians, and sometimes teachers. Dr. Miller perceived John Shaw Billings (1838-1913) as one of the most productive and creative of those individuals. She also saw him as a transition figure who helped pave the way for the Garrisons, Sigerists, and other more or less full-time medical historians. In this paper, I will elaborate upon and extend some of Dr. Miller's findings about Billings. In particular, I want to bring out the reasons why and how Billings deliberately limited his activities as a medical historian, thus remaining a part-time contributor to that scholarly field despite opportunities to devote himself exclusively to it.

Apart from Dr. Miller, medical historians have seldom recognized or written about John Shaw Billings's historical pursuits. One major reason for this neglect has been that those activities had unfolded largely in the context of Billings's incredibly broad scientific and professional life, and were inevitably overshadowed by the extensive attention given to the various facets of that life. Speakers at his 1913 memorial services recalled some of the highlights: his career up to 1895 as an innovative military surgeon; the pioneering medical library that he had built for the Army; his design of the Johns Hopkins Hospital; his gargantuan labors for the National Board of Health, his collaboration with Herman Hollerith to develop tabulating machines for the United States Census; and, later on, his shaping of such nonmedical landmarks as the New York Public Library and the Carnegie Institution of Washington.

None of the memorial speakers praised or apparently even remembered Billings as having been an historian. Those who did remember doubtless marveled that he had ever found time for the study of history. Yet, up to 1895 he did make time for it, at least sporadically. In fact, during those years, with other like-minded medical scientists, he came to be guided by the assumption that the insights of medical historical studies were or could be little if any less important than the insights from scientific study or laboratory research, at least in the long run. And as this conviction strengthened, it gave force to his initiatives to build up medical history resources or pursuits both for the Army and for the Johns Hopkins University. My remarks, therefore, will mainly divide into two parts focusing respectively on those institutions.

The Billings who joined the staff of Surgeon General Joseph Barnes late in the Civil War was still only twenty-six years old and apparently had no special medical history interests as yet. But he did have a deep-seated propensity for book learning in general. He thus seems to have pricked up his ears when Barnes began to talk about the possibility of creating a proper medical library for the

Army. In the late 1860s, when Barnes decided to go ahead with the project, he appointed Billings to direct it. Over the next quarter of a century, despite periodic changes of Surgeons General, Billings remained in charge of the library, which he energetically fashioned into an important and remarkably successful medical institution. Clearly, his increasing involvement in medical history could hardly have occurred but for this extended tour of library duty in Washington.

Billings's appointment as director of the Library did not include an explicit mandate to be a historian as well. However, the position did require him to take active roles in certain library functions that were partly or indirectly historical in nature. The collecting function, for one, took Billings into a fiercely competitive world that included businessmen as well as rare book librarians, historical scholars as well as dealers. By the 1880s, for instance, he was dickering with the book collector John Stockton Hough over potential additions to the Library's collection of medical incunabula. And beginning earlier, he started carrying on a vigorous program of exchanging duplicate works, both old and new, with Harvard's James Read Chadwick and other like-minded medical librarians.

Another library service that appealed to Billings was the extending of research assistance to individual scholars. As more historically interested physicians and scientists became aware of the historical resources of the Library, Billings satisfied as many of their requests for loans as he could. At the same time, he gained plaudits for his willingness to help find answers to their questions. For instance, when George Engelmann, Jr., of St. Louis, sought assistance in preparing an article on the history of obstetrics, Billings replied promptly and at some length. He could not, of course, perform the actual research and writing for the other man, but as usual he drew together for him an extensive reading list on the subject. Moreover, he promised that, if Engelmann could arrange to come to Washington for a week, Billings and his colleagues would place the Library's collections at the other's disposal and help guide his research.

Before that, in 1881, the Montreal clinician William Osler had already made his own initial two-day visit to the Library. Billings and his assistant Robert Fletcher, true to form, took time out to show him around, particularly among the older works of the collection. This visit led to a permanent friendship between the three men and to their close collaboration in several facets of late nineteenth-century medicine. At an early date, Billings also gave Osler borrowing privileges in the Library, and began as well to send him copies of the Library's publications. In turn, Osler reciprocated handsomely, first by sending Billings duplicate copies of books from his own library and later searching for copies of past Canadian institutional literature, including old medical college catalogs, health department and hospital reports, and other documents.

One of the largest library tasks for Billings, one that he began working on in the early 1870s, was that of preparing or supervising the preparation of specialty bibliographies and other finding guides to the institution's collections. He started with his large bibliography of cholera in 1875, and shortly afterward committed the Library almost in perpetuity to the indexing and publishing of its entire constantly growing bibliographical record. The two segments of that enterprise, of course, the *Index Catalogue* and the *Index Medicus* proved to be the principal ingredients in the library's success, but not the only ones. Over the years, Billings compiled other short guides, including his 1894 bibliography on the medical effects of alcohol. Moreover, he used some of the guides as partial models for two of the relatively small number of his personal historical publications.

The first of these was a long article that he wrote for the *American Journal of the Medical Sciences* to help mark the one hundredth anniversary of the country's independence. The article was basically a bibliographical summary of selected historical holdings that were already in the library, though Billings enhanced the interest of some of the entries with his personal comments. In his introduction, he described the work simply as a collection of "statistics obtained from a nearly complete list of the medical books published in this country from 1776 to the present time," together with data pertaining to medical societies, libraries, journals, and schools. Really an annotated historical directory, it made no pretense to be a learned historical analysis. And it served its patriotic purposes in an effective and matter-of-fact way, without resorting to flag-waving. Moreover, largely by inference, it also identified a considerable range of medical needs and targets to be expected in America's present and future.

Some twenty years later Billings issued a larger finding guide for another segment of the library's historical collections. Though ambitiously entitled the "History and Literature of Surgery," this work was much like its predecessor in format. It was really a factual listing of the surgeons, operations, and surgical publications of the past rather than a reasoned historical interpretation of that particular medical branch over time. The historian Fielding H. Garrison, writing after Billings's death, had mixed views about the publication as a contribution to history. Substantively, he considered it "the best work on the subject in English," and observed that it displayed a "genuinely critical spirit." At the same time, however he thought that potential readers must often have been turned off by its mode of presentation. Its long lists of obscure and unimportant names, in particular, made for "a certain dryness." Summing up, Garrison thought it a pity that Billings had chosen this unappealing bibliographical format when his usual personality was that of a "breezy spirit."

Billings's rapid build-up of the historical resources of the Surgeon General's Library, together with his production of bibliographical tools for the Library's historically minded readers, was nearly paralleled, timewise, by the emergence of opportunities for him to make major medical historical contributions outside the Army. This became possible in 1876, when the Surgeon General made him available as a part-time expert to help launch two large segments of Baltimore's new Johns Hopkins University. In one of these, as planner and medical advisor to the trustees of the Johns Hopkins Hospital, he shaped and brought that large building through to completion in 1889. At the same time, the University's President, Daniel Coit Gilman, invited Billings to be his principal consultant in planning and launching the medical school. This also proved to be a protracted process, one that occupied both men for the next decade and a half. While they had their differences in this venture, they shared a general desire to create a model medical school, one that would be closely integrated with the hospital, committed to the research ideal, and receptive to innovative educational methodologies.

To start his work for Gilman, Billings prepared and in 1877 presented a unique and highly crucial academic course. This was a series of twenty lectures that were intended to stimulate support for the new medical school among the university trustees and faculty, as well as among Baltimore physicians and the public. As justification for what was clearly to be a radical school, Billings drew extraordinarily heavily from the historical record. In fact, he devoted thirteen of his twenty lectures to a comprehensive review of the medical lessons of the past. Eleven of them covered the historical roots of western medicine and medical education from antiquity through the eighteenth century, while two others dealt with the early United States. Four lectures were then devoted to reviewing the existing medical schools, medical legislation, and related matters in mid-nineteenth century Europe, while three concluding lectures provided the details of Billings' recommendations as to "the Course to be pursued by the Hopkins University."

The course of twenty lectures was presented in a rented hall in Baltimore as one of the earliest academic events of the new university. For Billings, the writing of the lectures was a tour de force, carried out at white heat in a remarkably short time. They could not have been prepared at all without his easy access to the holdings of the Surgeon General's Library.

Billings's biographers have concluded that here, as in other public appearances, he made an excellent impression as a speaker and that he was forceful, direct, and fluent in style. They have, however, given surprisingly little attention to the scholarly content and quality of the thirteen historical lectures, considered as a unit, even though it constituted one of the most comprehensive American reviews of the world's history of medicine undertaken up to that time. Sanford Larkey, who examined the presentations in manuscript form, used far more of his short 1938 commentary on the lectures to assert Billings' greatness as a historian than to analyze the lectures' intellectual substance. He did, however, find the lectures to be engaging in their narrative style and competent in fitting the details of medical history together chronologically.

Fielding H. Garrison, considering these historical lectures in 1915, found them "carefully prepared" and deserving of being published as a monograph. He seems to have found no sign of the arid bibliographical format that bothered him about some of Billings's other historical works. And substantively, he was impressed that the lectures reflected the German historical medicine of the day. However, Garrison did not specify any particular scholar who may have influenced Billings in this respect. An interesting hypothetical case might be argued that historian Herbert Baxter Adams, whom Gilman had brought to Hopkins at the same time as Billings, could have exerted such influence. But, I have found no specific evidence to support the notion of any direct influence by Adams or any other general historian.

Whatever intellectual influences to which he may have been exposed, Billings, as he began the project, did not believe that he would be able to produce anything of much originality or intellectual merit in the short time available. Recognizing this, he warned Gilman in 1876 not to expect anything of very high caliber. Rather, he perceived the historical lectures he was working up as being commonplace in nature, aimed mainly at medical men, and divested "of all technicalities." As he proceeded with the work, he became increasingly dissatisfied with this approach and regretted not having been able to prepare a different type of lecture series. He became convinced that a series on what he called the "philosophy of the history of medicine," and which, by blending medical knowledge with that of philosophy, government, science, and religion, for instance, would clearly make for "a higher and better type of [historical] work." Realistically, however, Billings was forced to conclude that he himself could never find the time needed for writing such a work. "I could only do it by putting about a year's reading and reflection into each lecture, since I must know much besides Medicine, to do it."

Billings thus refused to consider publishing the completed historical lectures unless some unlikely opportunity to drastically rewrite them presented itself. As he reminded Gilman, there was already an overabundance of uninspired writings on the subject, "mostly copied one from another, even as these lectures must be in the main." Accordingly, when he finished presenting the course, these particular manuscripts were filed away in Billings's office, virtually in limbo so far as Gilman and the university were concerned. Apparently, no steps were taken to ask Billings to give his original history of medicine lectures again, let alone to prepare and deliver a different course. And he himself was not about to volunteer.

On the contrary, about this time Billings drew a line as to how much history he could or wanted to fit in. With his heavy load of scientific and medical undertakings, he remained far too extended in the years after 1877 to think of keeping his medical-historical initiatives at Hopkins going on a regular or even frequent basis. Clearly, his main commitments with Hopkins itself were to get the hospital and medical school built. To help spread knowledge about the latter project and to expedite the planning for it during this period, Billings and Gilman thus decided to publish an edited version of Billings's last three public lectures, those nonhistorical presentations that contained his detailed proposals for the school. Moreover, in 1883, in order to extend and formalize Billings's advisory role to the medical school, Gilman appointed him lecturer in hygiene, one of its first five faculty members.

During the ensuing period, before the school was ready to accept regular students, the faculty was well aware that Billings's overall recommendations in 1877 had included the eventual provision of some sort of substantial academic program in the history of medicine. His justification of this revolutionary proposal was fairly concise. In the case of "ordinary" medical schools, Billings was certain that special programs in medical history would not be appropriate, since most of the students who went to such institutions planned to become general medical practitioners and simply did not have the time for very much exposure to history. For the Hopkins medical school, however, the circumstances were expected to be entirely different. Billings anticipated that much of its student body would be composed of individuals planning to teach, write, or carry on research. Accordingly, courses in medical history would be essential for them, not only as a "stimulus to thought" but in providing a "means of culture." These courses, of course, would need to be supplemented by thorough instruction in bibliographical methods. For such methodology, he saw, would be prerequisite to the competent ultimate functioning of the well-trained medical historian, whether he was doing research into the roots of past medical innovations or tracing the replications of erroneous medical theories and practices over the centuries.

Not surprisingly, Billings's medical history proposal had little chance of gaining much priority during the Hopkins Medical School's organizational period. Billings himself never seems to have expressed interest in playing a permanent academic role in bringing it about. And, apart from him, there was no other commanding figure or scholar in the United States who could organize and take over such a program. There were also few anywhere else. Moreover, in 1892, when the Medical School finally opened, it had no visible means of financing such a program. Nevertheless, possibly in the hope that Billings might ultimately help launch it, the school appointed him to a lectureship in the History and Literature of Medicine, one that he retained until 1905. Actually, however, during that period he never found time to present a full course of lectures in any one year, and only rarely gave more than three lectures.

For some time after 1905, the Johns Hopkins school failed to find anyone to continue the history of medicine lectureship. However, Billings's vision of a substantial, professionally based program or department for the subject, though quiescent, was somehow kept alive in the School, at least in the spacious mind of William H. Welch. And ultimately it came to fruition with the buildup of the Institute of the History of Medicine in the 1920s and 1930s.

Meanwhile, Billings's innovations at the nascent Johns Hopkins Medical School were attracting attention elsewhere. For a time, in fact, individuals at two other educational institutions tried to enlist Billings to do something in medical history for them. In 1886, Henry P. Bowditch invited him to present a series of six lectures on the subject at the Harvard Medical School. However, the two were apparently unable to agree upon dates; at least, I have found no record that

Billings ever delivered such a series at Harvard. Possibly to take their place, he shortly agreed to present a series of eight public lectures on medical history at the Lowell Institute of Boston. Apparently basing these at least to some extent upon his 1877 lectures, he seems to have delivered all eight by early 1888. However, only the first of them, the one dealing with the medical concepts of primitive peoples, was ever published. Once again, presumably, he was unable or unwilling to find the time necessary to put the other seven lectures into a historiographical and literary shape that he or an editor could accept.

In 1889, medical history in the Johns Hopkins community itself took a new turn with the opening of the hospital and the arrival of Osler. Billings, of course, was one of the members of the top-level Hopkins cabal that lured Osler away from the University of Pennsylvania. The plotters had also included President Gilman, Dean William H. Welch, and Francis T. King, head of the hospital board. Officially, they wanted Osler for two positions, as Physician in Chief of the hospital and as Professor of the Theory and Practice of Medicine in the medical school. But it was never much of a secret that, with the acquisition of Osler, Hopkins was also getting a competent though still part-time medical historian. And Billings, as he ended his tour as the hospital's medical advisor, was well satisfied with this arrangement.

With Osler aboard, then, the hospital and ultimately the medical school personnel began to get exposure to medical history on a virtually continuing basis. In his clinical teaching, Osler not only introduced substantive historical material into his presentations but involved his students in the process of searching for original medical-historical sources. At the same time, with Howard A. Kelly, Welch, and others, he organized the Johns Hopkins Hospital Historical Club, whose monthly meetings generated much interest among faculty and students alike.

Invited to become an honorary member of the Club, Billings went up from Washington for the meetings when he could, and sometimes he presented short papers or commentaries. On occasion, he would bring along one or more of the rare medical books that he had just acquired for the Surgeon General's Library. And with these impressive physical evidences of the past in hand, he would deliver short bibliographical descriptions of the tomes, summaries of the lives and times of the authors, and perceptive interpretations of the medical contents. Not a few members of the club, particularly those who were book collectors, are on record as having been influenced as much by these informal but knowledgeable presentations by Billings, as they were by the more finished and literary historical profiles that Osler tried out on the club members.

Billings himself enjoyed the meetings of the historical club as much as anyone. He was comfortable being with Welch, Osler, and other like-minded faculty members who participated. These were, of course, occasions when they could bask in the early fruits of the idealistic medical ambiance that they had been creating. Moreover, in their own ways, they took satisfaction in being surrounded by medical students, particularly at the point when the latter were beginning their attempts to augment their understanding of current medicine by their studies of medical history.

After Billings retired from the Army and moved to New York City, most of his previous involvements in medical history came to an end. At the New York Public Library, he found neither time nor opportunity for substantial personal initiatives in this field of study. And, for the most part, the same was true in his capacity as an official of the Carnegie Institution. However, his co-sponsorship of that institution's Department of Historical Research did associate him significantly with what was a pioneering foundation commitment of funds to stimulation the elevation of history in the United States.

Also in New York, during the years after 1898, some modest aspects of Billings's past career as a historian were recreated when he became a member of the recently established Charaka Club. Membership in that organization was composed of physicians, including such personal friends as Osler, Pearce Bailey, George F. Shrady, S. Weir Mitchell, and others, who met socially and gave occasional short papers to each other on the literary, artistic, and historical aspects of medicine. The club's meetings had already taken on an easy-going and undemanding character, apparently due to an implicit agreement of the members to deliver papers that would be interesting to their colleagues rather than aiming to impress by the depth of their scholarship. The club thus offered a relaxed and encouraging environment for those physicians who had only limited time for the pursuit of medical history. For Billings, at any rate, that seemed to be an ideal arrangement in the early twentieth century.

Selected Readings

1. Miller, Genevieve. In Praise of Amateurs: Medical History in America be fore Garrison. *Bul Hist Med* 47:586-615, 1973.

2. Garrison, Fielding H. *John Shaw Billings, A Memoir*. New York, G. P. Putnam's Sons, 1915.

3. Chapman, Carleton B. *Order Out of Chaos: John Shaw Billings and America's Coming of Age*. Boston, Boston Medical Library, 1994.

4. Harvey, A. McGehee and Abrams, Susan. John Shaw Billings: Unsung Hero of Medicine at Johns Hopkins. *Maryland His. Mag* 84:119-134, 1989.

5. Larkey, Sanford V. John Shaw Billings and the history of medicine. *Bull Hist Med* 6:360-376, 1938; and Larkey, Sanford V, Two letters by John Shaw Billings on the history of medicine," *Bull Hist Med* 6:394-398, 1938.

The Evolution of the Controlled Clinical Trial*

Sir Richard Doll

In 1950, **Richard Doll**, with Austin Bradford Hill (1897-1991), published in the *British Medical Journal* the first study linking the marked increase in lung cancer with cigarette smoking (*BMJ* 2:739-748, 1950). Since that time he has published a number of articles demonstrating the relation of smoking to lung cancer and other diseases. As one of the world's leading epidemiologists, he has contributed to our understanding of the causes of childhood cancer, the dose-response relations of ionizing radiation to cancer, the long-term effects of oral contraceptives, and the occupational hazard of asbestos.

Sir Richard Doll qualified in medicine at London University in 1937, worked as a physician full-time until 1945 and part-time until 1969, and served in the Royal Army Medical Corps in France and the Middle East, 1939-1945.

He began epidemiological research with Dr. Avery A. Jones in 1946, transferred to the Medical Research Council's Statistical Research Unit under Professor A. Bradford Hill in 1948, and was director of the unit from 1961-1969. From 1969-1979 he was Regius Professor of Medicine at the University of Oxford, and from 1970-1983 Warden of Green College, Oxford. Since 1983 he has been an honorary member of the Imperial Cancer Research Fund's Cancer Studies Unit. He was elected a Fellow of the Royal College of Physicians in 1956, a Fellow of the Royal Society in 1966, and foreign member of the National Academy of Sciences (USA) in 2001.

Professor Doll has served on many bodies including the UK Medical Research Council, the Scientific Council of the International

*Delivered 23 May 2003 at the Thirdy-third Annual Meeting of the American Osler Society, Edinburgh, Scotland.

Agency for Research on Cancer and the World Health Organization's Advisory Committee on Medical Research, and its Committee on Health and the Environment, and is currently Chairman of the Management Committee of the UK Childhood Cancer Study and the National Radiological Protection Board's Advisory Committee on Non--ionizing Radiation.

He has received honorary degrees from fourteen universities and many awards, including the United Nations Award for Cancer Research, 1962, the Charles S. Mott Prize for Cancer Research, 1979, the Prince Mahidol Award, 1992, the gold medal of the European Cancer Society, 2000, and the Tyler Prize for Environmental Achievement, 2003. In 1966 he received the Order of the British Empire, in 1971 he was knighted, and in 1996 he was made a Companion of Honour.

Introduction

When, in September last year, I was invited to give the McGovern lecture to the joint meeting of the Osler Societies of America and Japan and the Osler Club of London, I had to accept. For it was not only an honour that I greatly appreciated, but it also gave me an opportunity to acknowledge the debt that Green College, Oxford, and the Oxford Medical School both owe to Dr. McGovern and Oslerians worldwide. And our debt is great; for it is measured not only in the financial terms that have enabled 13 Norham Gardens to be maintained in part as a memorial to Sir William, housing a collection of Osleriana; but also in intellectual terms, as it has strengthened our capacity for teaching that the practice of medicine is not just the mechanistic process of diagnosis and prescription, but requires a sympathetic ear and an understanding of a patient's concerns. I have, as must be only too obvious, been retired from any responsibility for either the College or the Medical School for more years than I care to think, but I know I speak for both when I say that the help of Dr. McGovern and the continued interest of Oslerians are both greatly appreciated.

Origin of Controlled Trials

The subject that I have chosen for my talk is not one that might appear at first glance to be of great historical interest, but I hope I can persuade you that it is and that those who took the first steps towards the development of what is now an essential element of medical science should be better known than they are. For many doctors, I suspect, the concept of the controlled trial would be dated to the origin of the Medical Research Council's trial of streptomycin in the treatment of pulmonary tuberculosis in 1946, when Bradford Hill persuaded his clinical colleagues to allocate the new treatment to patients by some system of randomization,[1] and that little or nothing has happened since to modify its original form. Both beliefs are incorrect. The practicality, need for, and essential characteristics of the modern controlled trial had, in fact, been debated and even tentatively tested progressively over at least three centuries,[2] and several major changes have been made in the last fifty years to the 1946 model. The evolution of the trial has, in truth, been a slow and continuing process, which was speeded up in 1946, just as the evolution of *homo sapiens* that has occurred over several million years may have been qualitatively changed by a mutation in a single gene (protocadherin XY) that facilitated the development of language about 100,000 to 150,000 years ago.[3]

Initially, new treatments were introduced on the basis of trial and error by leaders of the profession who may have acted on theory or adopted folk remedies, and whose improved results, if indeed they were improved, were generally obtained by the displacement of harmful or more harmful remedies or by the psychotherapeutic effect of their personal attention and the treatments were subsequently used on the strength of their teaching.

Van Helmont's Proposal

The first conscious step of which we have record towards ensuring what we should now consider the essential prerequisite of a valid trial: namely, the elimination of bias in the selection of cases for comparison, was taken by John Baptista Van Helmont, a Flemish physician who challenged the orthodoxy of the day in the first half of the seventeenth century,

> If ye speak truth, Oh ye Schooles", he wrote, "that ye can cure any kinde of Fevers without evacuation, but will not fear of a worse relapse; come down to the contest ye Humorists. Let us take out of the Hospitals, out of the Camps, or from elsewhere, 200 or 500 poor people, that have Fevers, Pleurisies, etc. Let us divide them in halves, let us cast lots, that one half of them may fall to my share and the other to yours. I will cure them without bloodletting and sensible evacuation; but do you do as ye know (for neither do I tye you up to the boasting, or of Phlebotomy, or the abstinence from a solutive Medicine) we shall see how many Funerals both of us shall have. But let the reward of the contention, or wager, be 300 Florins, deposited on both sides. Here your business is decided.[4]

A fine offer indeed, but there is no record that it was ever taken up. Nor is it clear whether the toss of a coin was to decide who would get each member of a pair of patients, or whether this was to be decided by alternation or some other pseudorandom method and the toss of a coin was to decide which group Van Helmont was to treat—so-called cluster randomisation—but it was certainly an impressive proposal that would have eliminated the bugbear of many comparisons that continued to be made into the twentieth century: namely, the selection of a group of patients with a relatively good prognosis to test the investigator's favoured method.

Lind and the Treatment of Scurvy

It was in the UK, however some one hundred years later that the realisation of the need to compare like with like began to be taken seriously, epitomised by Lind's study of the comparative values of the various treatments recommended for scurvy, that was such a terrible hazard of long voyages to distant parts of the world in ships that carried little or no fresh food.[5] When Lind carried out his famous study he had no formal medical qualification (although he did obtain one later in Edinburgh) and had been only an apprentice to a local surgeon before becoming a surgeon in the navy.[5] In this capacity he had obtained a strong impression of the value of citrus fruits. He was not the first to think that they might be effective—Vasco da Gama's sailors are reported to have demanded oranges on their way back from India 250 years earlier, having seen their beneficial effect when stopping at Mombasa on their way out,[6] but he set out to test his impression scientifically by comparing their effect with that of five other treatments given under similar conditions. In his own words,

> On the 20th May, 1747, I took twelve patients in the scurvy on board the Salisbury at sea. Their cases were as similar as I could have them. They all in general had putrid gums, the spots and lassitude, with weakness of their knees. They lay together in one place, being a proper apartment of the sick in the fore-hold; and had one diet common to all, viz. water-gruel sweetened with sugar in the morning; fresh mutton-broth often times for dinner; at other times puddings, boiled biscuit with sugar, etc.; and for supper, barley and raisins, rice and currants, sago and wine, or the like.[7]

He then gave five pairs of patients five common treatments for a fortnight and the sixth pair two oranges and a lemon a day for six days before supplies ran out, and found that the last pair showed the most improvement, one sailor even becoming fit for duty.

The account of Lind's experiment was published as a treatise in Edinburgh in 1753,[7] but it was forty-two years before the Admiralty sanctioned the general use of lemon juice as a prophylactic against scurvy aboard its ships—a year after Lind had died. This is not the place to analyse the reasons for the delay, which were complex and, for the most part, not attributable to administrative incompetence[5] for I have cited Lind's experiment only as an illustration of the changing attitude to dogmatism and empiricism which marked British medicine in the second half of the eighteenth century and there were other claims of effective remedies to be taken into account.

Introduction of Alternation

In this period an increasing number of doctors in Britain began to demand numerical analysis of what actually happened to groups of patients diagnosed with different diseases and treated by different methods, rather than detailed accounts of the characteristics and progress of individual patients.[5] None, I regret to say, had any connection with Oxford, for the enthusiasm for science that led Oxford physicians and natural philosophers to found the Royal Society in the second half of the seventeenth century had waned and the leaders of the movement came, almost to a man, from Edinburgh. Many of them too were military or naval officers. Not having the social status within the medical hierarchy that Louis achieved in Paris a century later,[8] their work has been largely forgotten and the precedent for insisting on numerical analysis has been attributed to Louis. The records the Edinburgh physicians obtained had, however, revealed the high mortality associated with the customary practice of treating fever by 'anti-inflammatory evacuation' (that is bleeding, giving emetics, and purging) compared with reliance on cordials or the newly introduced cinchona bark, and prepared the way for an experiment in which different treatments were allocated alternatively without any selection by the investigator. The first such study, according to, Milne and Chalmers[9] was a study of the effect of bleeding by Alexander Hamilton and two other Army Surgeons that was conducted in a military hospital in Spain in the course of the war against Napoleon and was reported in Hamilton's doctoral thesis for the University of Edinburgh in 1816.[10] According to Hamilton,

> It had been so arranged that this number [that is 366 sick soldiers] was admitted alternately in such a manner that each of us had one third of the whole. The sick were indiscriminately received, and were attended as nearly as possible with the same care and accommodated with the same comforts. One third of the whole were soldiers of the 61st Regiment, the remainder of my own (the 42nd Regiment). Neither Mr Anderson nor I ever once employed the lancet. He lost two, I four cases; whilst out of the other third (treated with bloodletting by the third surgeon) thirty-five patients died.[10]

Twenty or so years later, according to West,[11] Balfour, another military surgeon with Edinburgh training, carried out a study in which alternation was used to test the efficacy of a claim that very small homeopathic doses of belladonna could prevent scarlet fever, then a serious life-threatening disease in children. "There were," Balfour reported,

> . . . 151 boys of whom I had tolerably satisfactory evidence that they had not had scarlatina. I divided them in two sections taking them alternately from the list, to prevent the imputation of selection. To the first section (76) 1 gave belladonna, to the second (75) I gave none; the result was that two in each section were attacked by the disease. The numbers are too small to make any deduction as to the prophylactic power of belladonna, but the observation is good because it shows how we are misled by imperfect observation. Had I given the remedy to all the boys I should probably have attributed to it the cessation of the epidemic.

If he had not succeeded in proving, or disproving the efficacy of belladonna as a prophylactic, Balfour had at least demonstrated his own scientific competence in both experimental design and in the interpretation of experimental results.

By the end of the century, alternation had evidently come to be accepted by many leading medical scientists as a standard method of investigation. When, for example, it came to introducing the new anti-toxin treatment for diphtheria, the Danish physician Johannes Fibiger (1898) wrote,

> In many cases a trustworthy verdict can only be reached when a large number of randomly selected patients are treated with the new remedy and, at the same time an equally large number are treated as usual. . . . I suggested to Professor Sørensen to treat all patients admitted on the one day with serum, but none of those who were admitted the following day.[12]

Delayed Medical Response

Despite these good examples, the fact is that as late as the 1930s, when I was a medical student in London, most new treatments were still introduced on the authority of professors or, in the UK, where there were few medical professors, that of eminent consultants, who compared the results they obtained in a series of patients with the, almost inevitably, less favourable results that others or they themselves had obtained previously. Sir William Osler relied on such methods himself; but he used them so perceptively that one of his great contributions was to discourage the use of 'nauseous mixtures' and to stress that there was an inherent tendency for many diseases to recover independently of any treatment, as in the majority of cases nature alone was quite competent to restore the patient to health. He was, however, not averse to formal statistical analysis for, in welcoming Sir Almroth Wright's introduction of immunization against typhoid fever, he commented that "It is only by the statistical method that we are able to judge the results in practice," adding that "The new iatro-Mathematical school of Pearson and his scholars have made the profession cautious in drawing results from statistics, but in the matter under consideration the figures are, I believe trustworthy."[13] Osler came to know Greenwood, the leading British medical statistician of the time, and according to Rosser Matthews[14] Greenwood wrote to Pearson that Osler was attempting to persuade Johns Hopkins to set up a statistical department and was arranging a symposium at Oxford on 'Iatro-mathematics.'[15] I have not, however, been able to trace any comment by Osler on the way that trials should be conducted or the need for concurrent controls.

Old ways, in fact, died hard and Bradford Hill, one of Pearson's pupils, still had to lay stress on the importance of concurrent controls in his series of articles on statistics in medicine that appeared in the *Lancet* in 1937. These articles, written in simple English, without the use of mathematical formulae, and subsequently republished in book form[16] had an immense influence in the English speaking world on what was, in general, an innumerate profession and gave authority to the use of alternation as an appropriate statistical design.

Early Randomised Trials

By this time, however, some other scientists, stimulated, in all probability by Fisher's work in agricultural science[17] had already begun to think about the use of randomisation in clinical trials. To Fisher, randomisation was the prerequisite for a scientific estimate of the statistical significance of any difference in the results obtained by two treatments. Emphasizing what he had written previously, he reiterated in his 1935 text that "The purpose of randomisation . . . is to guarantee the validity of the test of significance, this test being based on an estimation of error made possible by replication."[18]

The first examples I know of the use of randomisation in clinical trials are two trials of the possible effect of irradiation with ultraviolet light to prevent the common cold, a rather unsatisfactory one by Dora Colebrook[19] on behalf of the Medical Research Council in the late 1920s, and a more satisfactory one by Doull et al.[20] at Johns Hopkins University a few years later. On the advice of Professor Lowell Reed, Doull et al.[20] drew up, in alphabetical order, a list of 373 volunteers from students or members of the staff of the School of Hygiene, and then Reed withdrew a die from a bag that contained 122 white die, 66 red die, and 185 black die, which had been thoroughly mixed in a sampling machine. A white die indicated that the next person on the list should be allocated one treatment a week, a red die that he or she should have two treatments a week, and a black die no treatment. The results, in accord with Colebrook's, sadly showed no benefit from treatment.

A few years later a similar technique was used by Theobald[21] at St. Mary Abbot's Hospital, where there was an obstetric unit affiliated with the London

Postgraduate Medical School, to test the ability of a combination of calcium lactate, vitamin A, and vitamin D to prevent toxaemia in pregnancy. This time women presenting at an antenatal clinic withdrew a bead from a box containing equal numbers of blue and white beads and, according to the colour, they either received the special prophylactic treatment or did not receive it. Only one hundred women participated and the number, Theobald thought, was regrettably small; but the results were nevertheless statistically significant, the women who received the supplements having fewer signs and symptoms suggestive of toxaemia than those who did not. This, he thought, indicated an inadequate level of nutrition, something which was then distressingly common among women in England. A further trial that used the toss of a coin to decide which of two treatments individuals should receive was described by Hinshaw and Feldman[22] but it must be doubted whether it was ever put into effect.[23]

Meanwhile, another form of randomisation had been reported by Amberson et al.[24] They divided twenty-four patients with pulmonary tuberculosis into two equal groups, the members of each group having been "individually matched" in pairs and then tossed a coin to decide which group should be given the newly acclaimed treatment of sodium gold thiosulphate—a procedure reminiscent of what Van Helmont had proposed 260 years before. Their technique of cluster randomization suffers, however, from two disadvantages: the virtual impossibility of truly being able to match cases and the lack of any means of measuring the relevant random error, because the effective sample size was only two.[25]

Streptomycin for Pulmonary Tuberculosis

It was not, however, until after the Second World War that a trial was carried out that put randomisation on the map and led to its progressive adoption throughout the world for testing the efficacy of new treatments: namely, the Medical Research Council's trial of streptomycin for the treatment of pulmonary tuberculosis, that was designed by Bradford Hill and conducted by Marc Daniels.[1] It was not the first such trial that Hill had designed, for one to test the efficacy of immunization against whooping-cough had been started on similar lines a few months earlier.[26] The results of the vaccine trial were, however, published later and were less dramatic in their impact. The streptomycin trial, which might at first sight have been thought unethical, had been ethical in Britain because the supply of streptomycin was so limited and, what little there was, was ear-marked first for conditions that were uniformly fatal: namely, miliary tuberculosis and tuberculous meningitis. The government, strapped for US dollars after the war, was unable to provide more than a small sum to purchase a supply of an expensive foreign drug that could be used for less uniformly fatal conditions. Participation in the trial consequently ensured all the patients of the best treatment currently available with the immediate opportunity of a hospital bed (then in short supply), and a 50 percent chance of getting in addition a promising new treatment not otherwise available.

To Bradford Hill, the value of randomisation was not, as it was to Fisher, a theoretical justification for the use of statistical tests of significance, but a practicable means of ensuring the absence of bias in the allocation of cases. For he had found, from practical experience, that the use of alternation had at times led to discrimination in deciding whether a patient was eligible for admission, the most seriously ill patients not being admitted to the group that was to receive the investigator's favoured treatment. Randomisation, after it had been decided that the patient was eligible for the trial, avoided this pitfall and the avoidance of bias is now considered the basic justification for its use; the statistical advantage over alternation that concerned Fisher being of little practical importance.

Randomisation for clinical trials was not uniformly accepted overnight, some clinicians arguing that it was inefficient, because it did not permit discrimination between patients that could benefit and those that could not. To this Hill (personal communication) used to reply "Tell me the criteria to distinguish such patients and we will build it into the trial." He never had any detailed response to his challenge, but it was always agreed that randomisation could be limited to patients within strata defined by the clinician as having different prognoses—if the clinician could, in fact, define them sufficiently clearly for general medical use. Gradually, however, the use of randomisation spread and it is now so broadly accepted that it is nearly always a necessary element of trials submitted to licensing authorities for the approval of new drugs.

Later Developments

Large Trials. Satisfactory though it was, the streptomycin trial was not the last word in trial design, for there have subsequently been two important developments. First, it has come to be realized that trials may need to be organized on a qualitatively larger scale. Although some of the early trials were collaborative, in that they required the participation of several specialist groups to obtain sufficient patients for the conduct of the trial, the total number of patients in any one trial was seldom more than a few hundred and often less. This was fine, if the benefit of the new treatment was much greater than that of the old, as was the case with the initial trial of streptomycin and has been for some of the trials of cortisone; but it certainly was not when one was dealing with a drug that reduced the fatality rate from say 12 to 10 percent—an unimportant gain in many instances, but important when the condition was as common as myocardial infarction. For a small gain from the treatment of a common condition may be socially more important than a large gain from the treatment of a rare condition. That it was practicable by international collaboration to carry out a trial on tens of thousands of patients rather than on a few hundred has been demonstrated by the ISIS (International Study of Infarct Survival) series of trials of therapy for myocardial infarction (*vide* *infra*) which have consequently obtained such clear evidence of several modest effects that it has changed medical practice and avoided many premature deaths worldwide.[27, 28]

Factorial Design. Such large trials are expensive and time-consuming and there is much to be gained from testing two or more therapies in the one trial. Fortunately, this was made possible by the factorial design that began to be introduced in the 1930s,[29] and was illustrated very clearly by Wilson and colleagues[30] in the mid-1940s when they sought to test simultaneously the separate effects of supplements of cysteine and of reduced dietary fat on the course of infective hepatitis. At that period the standard method used by the scientifically minded to test a new remedy was alternation of new and old therapies and Wilson et al.[30] consequently gave alternate patients a supplement of 5 g cysteine a day, giving alternate patients in each group either a low fat or a high fat diet. When, therefore, the patients given supplementary cysteine were compared with those not given it, each group had had comparable diets, half having had a high fat diet and half a low fat diet and the comparability held with regard to supplementary cysteine when they compared the patients on the two diets. They were thus able, with 103 patients, to show some possible benefit from cysteine in that jaundice, liver enlargement, and biliuria lasted for a shorter time than when it was not given, but that no benefit, judged by the same criteria, was obtained by reducing the fat in the diet.

Six years later, after the introduction of randomization, I was able to extend Wilson and colleagues' method to test, in one and the same trial, three therapies for gastric ulcer, by giving successive patients, in random order, one or other of the eight possible combinations of the three therapies (a, b and c; a and b; a and c; b and c; a alone; b alone; c alone; or none of them) and showed, as a result, that ulcers healed more quickly if patients were kept in bed in hospital than when they were ambulant at home, but that nothing was gained by medication with ascorbic acid or phenobarbitone.[31]

The same procedure has now been adapted to large trials but with a better system of randomisation, ensuring that no treating clinician can have any knowledge of what the next combination of treatments is likely to be. Two therapies were, for example, successfully tested in 17,000 patients with myocardial infarcts showing beneficial effects from both aspirin and streptokinase so clearly that in many countries medical practice was quickly altered and both therapies were adopted[27] and three therapies were tested a few years later in a trial in 58,000 patients, only one of which (an angiotensin converting enzyme inhibitor) proved to have any detectable benefit.[28]

The Future

By emphasizing the importance of really large trials to obtain clear and definitive results, I have not wished to imply that these are the acme of controlled trials at which their evolution ends. That trials could be conducted on tens of thousands of patients has been a major development is, I believe, evident; but that is not to say that small trials will not continue to have their place. On the contrary, new remedies will inevitably be tested first in small trials or, at best, in trials of medium size; but these should be made much more effective by the greater specificity that knowledge of molecular biology should make possible, even so effective that (dare I say it) we may, on some occasions, complete the circle and go back to the use of historical controls.

The introduction of imanitab mesylate, which inhibits the action of the specific tyrosine kinase that is the product of the chromosomal translocation that characterises chronic myeloid leukaemia, is a case in point. The effect on the progress of the leukaemia in a handful of patients was so dramatic that the drug went straight into clinical use from the trial designed to discover its most appropriate therapeutic dose[32] just as the sulphonamides and penicillin had done in the first half of the last century.

Envoi

But leaving the future aside, which is always uncertain to predict, the development that has already occurred is, to my mind, among the most important in the methodology of clinical research in the last one hundred years. In this account of it I have restricted myself to the development of the science and, for my knowledge of that, I have been deeply indebted to Sir Iain Chalmers, who has done more than anyone else since Bradford Hill to bring home to all sections of the medical profession the need to base their practice on reliable evidence of the balance of benefit and harm from what they do, something that is now enshrined in the work of the worldwide Cochrane Collaboration that Sir Iain initiated.[2] I have consequently said very little about the ethical considerations that necessarily accompany every new step in Medicine, and nothing at all about the growth of regulations that are progressively being attached to the allocation of funds for research. Both need much more thought than they appear to have had, if research in the public interest is to be continued, and their examination is best reserved for another occasion and another speaker with more of Sir William's scholarship, clarity of presentation, and power to persuade than I could possibly hope to achieve.

Acknowledgment

I am most grateful to Dr. David Wirt of Houston, Texas for the Reference to Osler's 1914 paper[13] and the correspondence from Dr. Matthews[14]and to Sir Iain Chalmers[2] for drawing my attention to the fund of information in the Lind Library that he has established.

References

1. Medical Research Council Streptomycin in Tuberculosis Trials Committee. Streptomycin treatment for pulmonary tuberculosis. *Brit Med J* 2: 769-782, 1948.
2. Chalmers, I. Comparing like with like: some historical milestones in the evolution of methods to create unbiased comparison groups in therapeutic experiments. *Int J Epidemiol* 30:1156-1164, 2001.
3. Sargent, C.A., Blanco, P., and Affara, N.A. Did the hominid-specific regions of X-Y homology contain candidate genes potentially involved in a critical event linked to speciation? In: *The Speciation of Modern Homo Sapiens.* Crow, T.J. (Ed.). Oxford, Oxford University Press, 2002.
4. Van Helmot, J.B. *Oriatrike, or Physick Refined: the Common Errors therein Refuted and the Whole Art Reformed and Rectified.* Translated by J.C. Sometime. London, Lodowick-Lloyd, 1662.
5. Tröhler, U. *"To improve the evidence of Medicine." The 18th century British origins of a critical approach.* Edinburgh, Royal College of Physicians of Edinburgh, 2000.
6. Alvaro Velho A., and Ravenstin R.G. *Journal of the First Voyage of Vasco da Gamo 1497-1499.* Columbia, South Asia Books, 1998.
7. Lind, J. A *Treatise of the Scurvy. In Three Parts. Containing an Inquiry into the Nature, Causes and Cure, of that Disease. Together with a Critical and Chronological View of what has been Published on the Subject.* Edinburgh, Printed by Sands, Murray and Cochran for A. Kincaid and A. Donaldson, 1753, pp. 145-146
8. Greenwood, M. *The Medical Dictator and Other Biological Studies.* London, Williams & Norgate, 1936.
9. Milne, I. and Chalmers, I. Tackling bias in assessing the effects of health care interventions: early contributions from James Lind, Alexander Lesassier Hamilton, and T. Graham Balfour. *Proc Royal Soc Edinburgh* 31(Suppl 9):46-48, 2001.
10. Hamilton, A.L. *Dissertatio Medica Inauguralis De Synocho Castrensi.* Edinburgh, J Ballantyne, 1816.
11. West, C. *Lectures on the Diseases of Infancy and Childhood.* London, Longman, Brown, Green and Longmans, 1854, p. 600.
12. Fibiger, J. Om serumbehandlung af Difteri. *Hospitalstidende* 6: 309-325, 337-350, 1898.
13. Osler, W. The war and typhoid fever. *Brit Med J* 2:909-913, 1914.
14. Mathews, J.R. Letter to Dr. Daniel P. Wirt (Wirt, personal communication).
15. Greenwood, M. On methods of research available in the study of medical problems, with special reference to Sir Almsroth Wright's recent utterances. *Lancet* 1: 164, 1913.

16. Hill, A.B. *Principles of Medical Statistics.* London, *Lancet*, 1937.
17. Fisher, R.A. *Statistical Methods for Research Workers.* Edinburgh, Oliver & Boyd, 1925.
18. Fisher, R.A. *The Design of Experiments.* Edinburgh, Oliver & Boyd, 1935.
19. Colbrook, D *Irradiation and Health.* London, Medical Research Council Special Report Series No. 131, 1929.
20. Doull, J.A., Hardy, M., Clark, J.H., and Herman, N.B. The effect of irradiation with ultraviolet light on the frequency of attacks of upper respiratory dis ease (common colds). *Am J Hyg* 13: 460-477, 1931.
21. Theobold, G.W. Effect of calcium and vitamins A & D on incidence of pregnancy toxaemia. *Lancet* 1: 1397-1399, 1937.
22. Hinshaw, H.C. and Feldman, W.H. Evaluation of chemotherapeutic agents in clinical tuberculosis: a suggested procedure. *Am Rev Tuberc* 50: 202-213, 1944.
23. Doll, R., Peto, R., and Clarke, M. First publication of an individually randomized trial. *Controlled Clinical Trials* 20:367-368, 1999.
24. Amberson, J.B., McMahon, B.T., and Pinner, M. A clinical trial of sanocrysin in pulmonary tuberculosis. *Am Rev Tuberc* 24: 401-435, 1931.
25. Armitage, P. The role of randomisation in clinical trials. *Statistics in Med* 1: 345-352, 1982.
26. Medical Research Council Whooping-cough Immunization Committee. The prevention of whooping-cough by vaccination. *Brit Med J* 1: 1463-1471, 1951.
27. ISIS-2 (Second International Study of Infarct Survival) COLLABORATIVE GROUP. Randomised trial of intravenous streptokinase, oral aspirin, both, or neither among 17,187 cases of suspected acute myocardial infarction: ISIS-2. *Lancet* 2: 349-360, 1988.
28. ISIS-4 (Fourth International Study of Infarct Survival) Collaborative Group. ISIS-4: A randomised factorial trial assessing early oral captopril, oral mononitrate, and intravenous magnesium sulphate in 58,050 patients with suspected acute myocardial infarction. *Lancet* 345: 669-685, 1995.
29. Doll, R. Controlled trials testing two or more treatments. In press.
30. Wilson, C., Pollock, M.R. and Harris, A.D. Diet in the treatment of infectious hepatitis. *Lancet* 1: 881-883, 1946.
31. Doll, R. and Pygott, F. Factors influencing the rate of healing of gastric ulcers: admission to hospital, phenobarbitone, and ascorbic acid. *Lancet* 1: 171, 1952.
32. Druker, B.J., Talpaz, M., Resta, D.J., Peng, B., Buchdunger, E., Ford, J.M., Lydon, N.B., Kantarjian, H., Capdeville, R., Ohno-Jones, S., and Sawyers, C.L. Efficacy and safety of a specific inhibitor of the BCR-ABL tyrosine kinase in chronic myeloid leukaemia. *N Engl J Med* 344: 1031-1037, 2001.

About the Editor

Lawrence D. Longo is Professor of Obstetrics and Gynecology, Physiology, and Biochemistry, School of Medicine, Loma Linda University, Loma Linda, California. Although working as a basic scientist, Dr. Longo has published a number of articles on nineteenth-century obstetrics and gynecology. In addition to several volumes on fetal physiology, Dr. Longo has published *A Short History of the Society for Gynecologic Investigation, 1953-1983* (1983); "Charles White and the Evolution of Ideas Concerning the Etiology and Prevention of Puerperal Fever"; Introduction to *A Treatise on the Management of Pregnant and Lying-in Women* by Charles White (1987); and with T.K.A.B. Eskes *Classics in Obstetrics and Gynecology, Innovative Papers That Have Contributed to Current Clinical Practice* (1993). His latest book, with Philip M. Teigen, is *"Dearest G . . ., Yours W.O.," William Osler's Letters from Egypt to Grace Revere Osler* (2002). Currently, he is completing a volume *Robert Patterson Harris of Philadelphia: The "Statistical Method" and the Evolution of Cesarean Section.*